*Collective Biographies*

# AIDS

## Ten Stories Of Courage

Doreen Gonzales

**ENSLOW PUBLISHERS, INC.**

44 Fadem Road      P.O. Box 38
Box 699      Aldershot
Springfield, N.J. 07081    Hants GU12 6BP
U.S.A.      U.K.

For their kind assistance in this project, I would like to thank Judy Burnett, Gary Shilts, Leslie Flores, Carol Gertz, Victoria Leacock, John Loengard, Cindy and Stewart Haskell, and Joe Amati.

**Library of Congress Cataloging-in-Publication Data**

Gonzales, Doreen.
        AIDS : ten stories of courage / Doreen Gonzales.
          p. cm.— (Collective biographies)
        Includes bibliographical references and index.
        Summary: Presents the stories of ten people who have been infected with AIDS, including Ryan White, Elizabeth Glaser, and Arthur Ashe.
        ISBN 0-89490-766-2
          1. AIDS (Disease)—Patients—Biography—Juvenile literature.
        2. Celebrities—Biography—Juvenile literature. [1. AIDS (Disease)—Patients.]
I. Title. II. Series.
RC607.A26G58 1996
362.1'969792'00922—dc20                 95-31115
[B]                                      CIP
                                              AC

Printed in the United States of America

10 9 8 7 6 5 4 3 2 1

**Illustration Credits:** The Ryan White Foundation, pp. 6, 13; Bettman, p. 23; MAH/Shooting Star, p. 16; Gary Shilts, p. 26; Leslie Flores, p. 31; Anonymous, pp. 43, 86; © 1990 John Loengard, p. 36; ©1994 The Estate of Keith Haring, pp. 46, 52; MIRA, p. 63; Martha Swope, p. 56; George Brick/Shooting Star, pp. 66, 72; Peter Hince/© Queen Productions Ltd. 1987, p. 76; Peter Hince/© Mighty Tape Ltd., 1987, p. 82; International Tennis Hall of Fame and Tennis Museum at The Newport Casino, Newport, Rhode Island, p. 91; Andrew D. Bernstein/NBA Photos, pp. 96, 101.

**Cover Illustration:** Mary Ann Carter

# Contents

# Preface

Over a quarter of a million Americans have died from AIDS, a disease brought on by a virus known as HIV. HIV is contracted when infected blood or sexual fluids are taken directly into an uninfected person's system. This most commonly occurs by having sex with an infected person, using an infected needle intravenously, or receiving blood from an infected person. An HIV-infected mother can also pass the virus to her child while she is pregnant or through her breast milk, when nursing her baby.

HIV does not care if a person is heterosexual, homosexual, bisexual, or celibate (having no sex at all). It does not look to see if a person is black or white, male or female, young or old. It does not ask a person's financial status, moral beliefs, or career path. The fact is, HIV simply invades any body it can, reproduces itself, and eventually kills.

Each of the thousands of people who have died from AIDS was a vital human being who loved, laughed, and had dreams for the future. Each suffered personal anguish at having life cut short. Some lived in fear of having their illness discovered by a disapproving society. Many endured intense physical pain. All left behind family and friends to whom they are irreplaceable.

Among these thousands were many who possessed outstanding talents which they used to touch lives beyond their personal acquaintances. Exceptional artists, athletes, scientists, writers, musicians, activists, and doctors, to name a few, have died of AIDS. In this book, ten famous people who have been stricken by AIDS are profiled. Each, by virtue of talent or circumstance, rose to prominence and made our lives better. From creative artist to committed activist to accomplished athlete, they demonstrate the breadth and depth of the talent AIDS has stolen from the world. These ten men and women are of varied ages, ethnicity, social strata, and sexual preference. Summarily, they represent us all. Because AIDS forever changed their lives, so too, it has forever changed ours.

The Center for Disease Control operates a telephone hotline that is open twenty-four hours a day, seven days a week. The counselors there are trained to answer questions regarding AIDS and HIV. These counselors can also help callers find other organizations that might assist them. All calls are free and anonymous.

CDC National AIDS Hotline
(800)342-2437

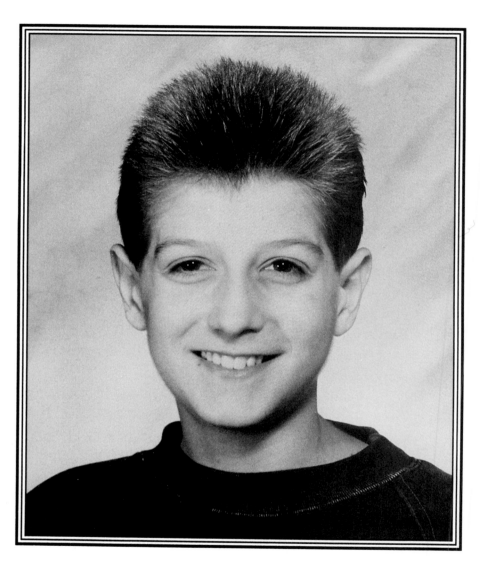

Ryan White

*During his short life on earth, Ryan touched millions of people, and I believe that in his new life he is doing the same. Ryan White was a miracle of humanity.*

—Elton John[1]

# Ryan White
## (1971–1990)

In many ways, Ryan White was just like other teenagers. He dreamed of getting his driver's license, loved junk food, and planned to go to college; but Ryan was different in one overwhelming, all-encompassing way. He had AIDS, a disease for which there is no known cure. Everyone who has ever had AIDS has died from it.

AIDS stands for Acquired Immune Deficiency Syndrome. It is brought on by a virus called human immunodeficiency virus (HIV). HIV makes its home in a person's blood where it may be inactive for years. Then one day it begins breaking down the body's immune system. Without a healthy immune system, the body has no defense against invading germs or diseases. When an HIV-infected person becomes ill with certain infections and cancers, he or she is said to have AIDS. AIDS patients eventually die of one or more of the illnesses that attack the weakened body. Ryan White knew this, but he tried not to worry about dying. He once said it was not how or when one dies that was important, but "how you live your life that counts."[2]

Ryan was born on December 6, 1971, in Kokomo, Indiana. He was the first child of Wayne and Jeanne White. Shortly after his birth, doctors discovered he suffered from hemophilia.

Hemophilia is another disease of the blood. Healthy blood contains clotting factors which stop bleeding when blood vessels break. The blood of a hemophiliac, however, does not have clotting factors. Instead, their blood accumulates inside the body, causing pain, swelling, and sometimes loss of function. Unchecked bleeding can even cause death. Although hemophilia cannot be cured, it can be treated by injecting the hemophiliac with the missing clotting factors, commonly called Factor.

Ryan's mother, Jeanne, wanted him to live as normally as possible. She felt confident that Factor could treat any injuries he might incur. So Ryan spent his early childhood like other youngsters—pedaling a toy car up and down the sidewalk, soaring high in a backyard swing, and climbing the tree in his grandparents' yard.

However, this was an unusually active life

for a hemophiliac. Before Ryan was five, he was treated at the hospital several times. There the doctors gave him Factor and occasional blood transfusions. During these visits, Ryan met children with illnesses more serious than his, so he rarely felt sorry for himself.

By the time Ryan entered school, Jeanne was giving him Factor at home each week. At about this time, his parents divorced. Ryan and his sister, Andrea, stayed with their mother and rarely saw their father.

Ryan was a good student. He tried to keep up with his classmates physically, but even with Factor, his blood did not always clot quickly and his legs and arms were frequently sore. However, he did not complain. When he was eight he insisted on playing Little League baseball and stuck with it through the summer. Later, two upsetting injuries convinced him to give up organized sports. Instead, Ryan spent his time collecting miniature cars and comic books. He also enjoyed fishing with his grandfather and biking around the neighborhood with friends. Later, Ryan would become an avid skateboarder.

Factor injections became a way of life for Ryan. Each one seemed much like another. In 1982, Ryan and his grandfather read about a new disease called AIDS. At the time, doctors did not know much about how AIDS was transmitted from one person to another. They did not fully understand that HIV could be transferred through the blood. They did know that some hemophiliacs were coming down with the disease.

This was because the Factor that hemophiliacs used was made from the blood of thousands of donors. If the blood of any one of these donors contained HIV, the entire batch of Factor would be contaminated and could pass the virus on to those who used it. Unfortunately, it was not until 1985 that donated blood was tested to see if it contained the HIV virus. In the meantime, Ryan had received hundreds of Factor injections.

During the autumn of 1984, Ryan started having diarrhea, stomach cramps, and night sweats. Tragically, doctors discovered he had a type of pneumonia common to people with AIDS. They then confirmed that Ryan had AIDS.[3] Because at least one of his Factor injections had been infected with HIV, Ryan entered his teenage years under a death sentence.

Grief-stricken, Jeanne gathered her strength and told her thirteen-year-old son that he had been infected. AIDS frightened Ryan. He wanted to pretend he did not have it. Then one night he dreamed he was making his way toward a brilliant light which he believed to be God. As he approached the light, God told him not to worry, that He would take care of him. When Ryan awoke, he was no longer afraid of death.

When the people in Kokomo heard that Ryan

had AIDS, they panicked. Fearing he might pass AIDS on to them, many of Ryan's neighbors and friends avoided him. Some of them even ran the other way when they saw him coming. At the time, AIDS was most common among homosexual men, and Ryan was called a "queer," "homo," and "faggot." The tires of the family car were slashed and Ryan's friends were prohibited from playing with him. In the summer of 1985, the school board banned Ryan from returning to school in the fall.

Jeanne was not sure Ryan should go to school, anyway. There, he would be exposed to all kinds of germs against which he had little resistance. Ryan, however, felt differently. Adamantly, he told his mother, "We *have* to fight, Mom. If we don't, we won't be allowed to go anywhere or do anything. What they want to do isn't right. We can't let it happen to anybody else."[4] So Jeanne fought to get Ryan readmitted to school. The Whites' lawsuit made national news and reporters from around the country poured into Kokomo to cover the story.

In April of 1986, Ryan won his case and returned to school only to encounter renewed attempts to make him leave. Students wrote obscenities on his locker and classmates taunted him. Ryan did his best to ignore the ugliness, but it was clear that he would never belong.

During the fall of 1986, AIDS illnesses kept

Ryan out of school. By January, he weighed only fifty-four pounds and was vomiting every twenty minutes. He was constantly cold and could keep his hands warm only by holding them over the burners of the electric stove. At the end of each day Jeanne prayed, "Thank you, dear Lord, for another day."[5] Ryan, too, felt that death was near.

One day, someone shot a bullet through the Whites' living room window. The Whites decided they had had enough—Ryan would not die in Kokomo. In May 1987, the family moved to the nearby town of Cicero, Indiana. To the Whites' happy surprise, the new neighbors greeted them warmly. The school's principal campaigned to welcome Ryan. He invited AIDS experts to speak with students and sent AIDS literature home. His efforts were effective and the community opened its arms to Ryan. This loving acceptance worked a magic on Ryan. His health improved dramatically and his spirits soared. Now he felt a calling to help others with AIDS. He had experienced the destructive power of ignorance, and was determined to prevent others from enduring the same misery.

On a personal mission to enlighten the country about AIDS, Ryan appeared on television shows and spoke to groups everywhere. He especially liked talking to children, feeling that they were better listeners than adults. Before long, Ryan was being called "one of the nation's most persuasive advocates for AIDS patients' rights."[6] He

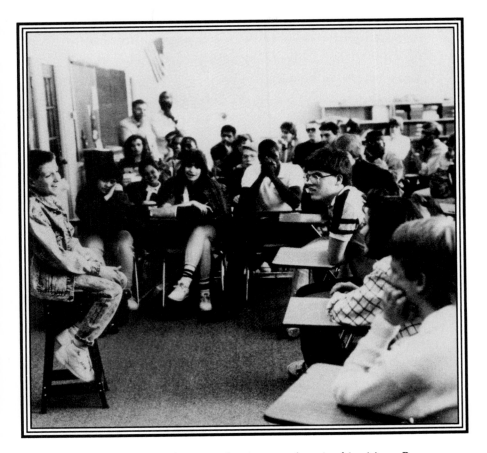

Ryan enjoyed speaking to other teens such as in this visit to Boys Town in Nebraska.

even testified before the Presidential Commission on AIDS.

The whole country was learning about Ryan White. Celebrities who were impressed with Ryan's message rallied to his cause. One, singer Elton John, became an especially close family friend and visited Ryan whenever he could.

Unfortunately, AIDS, too, was a frequent visitor. In March 1990, Ryan became so ill that he had to be hospitalized. His liver, spleen, and kidneys were shutting down, and his chances of surviving this attack were bleak. Ryan was only eighteen years old. For the first time ever, he said he was tired of fighting AIDS. Ryan agreed to be put on a ventilator to help him breathe. To do so meant having to be put under anesthesia, and Ryan knew he might never wake up.

For one week, Ryan lay unconscious while America watched and waited. As April 8 dawned, Jeanne, Andrea, Ryan's grandparents, and Elton John stood beside his bed. Filled with the deepest sorrow she had ever known, Jeanne leaned over her son and whispered, "Just let go, Ryan. It's all right, sweetheart."[7]

At 7:11 A.M. Ryan White died.

Fifteen hundred people gathered on April 11 to honor Ryan. During his funeral, the school choir sang "That's What Friends Are For," a song that was written to raise money for AIDS research. Elton John also sang. Jeanne White told mourners she wanted Ryan to be "remembered as somebody who accomplished a lot."[8]

With his smile that could light up a room, Ryan had indeed accomplished a lot. He had shown America AIDS through the eyes of a courageous and selfless child.

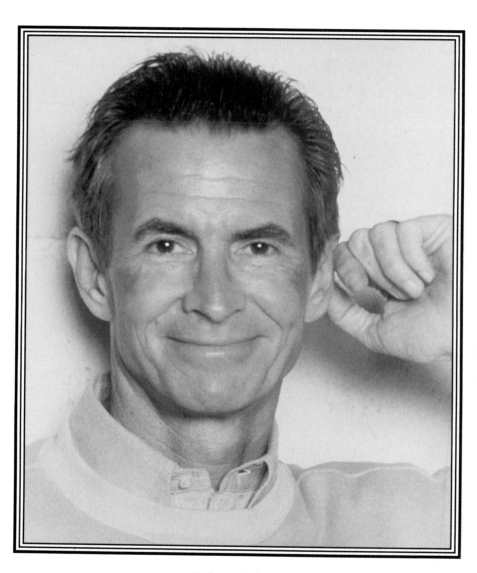

Anthony Perkins

# Anthony Perkins

## (1932–1992)

Norman seemed like such a nice young man. He took care of his ailing mother, ran the family business, and was kind to strangers. Or was he? There was something a bit disturbing about Norman Bates, something hard to define. In time, his bizarre peculiarity became apparent, and when it did, most people were glad that Norman Bates was only a character in a movie. Superbly played by actor Anthony Perkins, Bates seemed so real that he lived on in fiction for years after his first appearance in the 1960 horror movie classic, *Psycho*. But *Psycho* was only one of many movies in which Anthony Perkins proved to be a master actor.

Anthony Perkins was born in New York City in 1932, the only child of actor Osgood Perkins and Janet Rane. Young Anthony saw little of his father, who was frequently away making movies. As a result, he was especially close to his mother. When his father did come home, Anthony did not want to share his mother. "I loved [my father]," Anthony later said, "but I also wanted him to be dead so I could have [my mother] all to myself."[2] When Mr. Perkins had a heart attack and died suddenly, five-year-old Anthony was horrified. He believed that by wanting his father dead, he had actually killed him. A tremendous guilt settled on the boy and he spent many nights crying himself to sleep while praying for his father to come back.

Meanwhile, Anthony's relationship with his mother intensified. She smothered him with love and was overly attached to him. She seemed to rule his every action. As an adult, Perkins recalled, "She wasn't ill-tempered or mean. Just a strong-willed, dominant, New England kind of woman. She controlled everything about my life, including my thoughts and feelings."[3]

In addition, Mrs. Perkins told Anthony exaggerated stories about how wonderful his father had been. Other people, too, seemed to have adored Osgood Perkins. Deciding that he wanted this kind of admiration for himself, Anthony set out to be an actor—perhaps one even better than his father.

To that end, Anthony acted in every school play

and Sunday School pageant possible. When he was fourteen, he got a summer job acting. This led to other theater parts, and at sixteen Anthony was cast in a play that was going on tour.

After high school, Perkins spent three years at a small college in Florida, where he appeared in many plays. During one vacation, he hitchhiked to Hollywood. While watching a movie audition there, he was asked to read lines with someone who was trying out for a part. The director was so impressed with Perkins's reading that he hired him for a small part in a movie called *The Actress*.

This success gave Perkins confidence, so he transferred to Columbia University in New York City to be close to television studios. He earned several small roles in television dramas, then auditioned for a movie in 1953. Although he did not get the part for which he tried out, he was hired for a Broadway play called *Tea and Sympathy*. The show ran for more than a year. During this run, Perkins caught the eye of a few Hollywood directors, and his film career was off and running.

In Perkins's second movie, *Fear Strikes Out*, he played a Boston Red Sox outfielder battling a mental illness. In 1956, Perkins acted alongside movie legend Gary Cooper in a film called *Friendly Persuasion*, about a Quaker family during the Civil War. His performance as the son earned him a nomination for an Academy Award. More movies followed and Perkins was cast with stars such as Audrey Hepburn and Sophia Loren.

Then, in 1960, came *Psycho* and one of the most acclaimed roles of Perkins's acting career. Clearly, he had developed into the great actor he had hoped to become. However, while *Psycho* made him successful, it colored the way directors thought of him. All of the movie parts he now received seemed to be of mentally disturbed characters like Norman Bates. At thirty-four years old, Perkins was worried that he would be forever typecast. So he visited a psychotherapist to see if she could help.[4]

After the first few meetings, it was plain that Perkins' professional dilemma was secondary to his personal problems. Although he had hidden his feelings from others and even from himself, Perkins was still troubled by the events of his childhood. His mother's abnormal attachment to him had made him afraid of women. Even when he met beautiful actresses, he had no interest in dating them. So Perkins met with his therapist four times each week trying to resolve these troubles left over from childhood.

In time, Perkins grew more comfortable with women. One day he saw a picture of photographer Berry Berenson. He had never met her, but something about Berenson appealed to Perkins. Coincidentally, Berenson herself had been a Perkins fan when she was a teenager. She had kept scrapbooks of him from early movies and had often fallen asleep dreaming about him. As fate would have it, Perkins soon met Berenson at a party. She possessed a serenity that he found irresistible. The two began dating, fell in love, and were married in 1973.

Because Perkins wanted a healthy, happy family life, he continued his psychotherapy. Soon two sons, Osgood and Elvis, enlivened the Perkins' home. Perkins was an active, involved father—he changed diapers and refused jobs that would take him out of town. As his sons grew older, Perkins often made his boys breakfast and dinner and helped them with their homework. The family lived in a plainly furnished three-bedroom house and drove a Toyota station wagon. The Perkinses could have been any one of thousands of families across the United States.

Those closest to the family believed that Perkins had succeeded in his quest for a happy life. A longtime friend once remarked:

> I've read these stories about the disturbing psychological problems Tony had as a child, but you never saw them in that family. Every Christmas and Thanksgiving and Easter and New Year's we'd all go to Tony and Berry's. There was such love and such warmth, always. The Perkins home was where you came for family love. They're probably the happiest family I've known out here.[5]

Throughout these years, Perkins had been earning good parts in movies and plays. Among his many films were *Catch 22* (1970), *The Life and Times of Judge Roy Bean* (1972), and *Murder on the Orient Express* (1974). Later came three sequels to the original *Psycho* (1983, 1986, 1990). Between shows, the family's home was one of Perkins's favorite retreats. "He could spend days and days alone in this house, never want to get out, just putter around. He loved it," Berenson once said.[6]

Then, in 1990, came a terrible shock. An article in a supermarket tabloid claimed that Perkins was HIV-positive. Although Perkins himself had no knowledge of this, he immediately had himself tested. Tragically, it was true—he was carrying the HIV virus.[7]

How did the tabloid know about Perkins's infection? The family decided that the information might have arisen during Perkins's recent visit to a hospital for an unrelated problem. Devastated, Berenson immediately had herself and their sons tested. Finding that none of them was carrying the virus was a relief, but also baffling.

Just as baffling was how Perkins had contracted the HIV virus in the first place. The U.S. Department of Health and Human Services keeps statistics about how AIDS patients acquire the disease. Each year, hundreds of people report the source of their infection as unknown. Through lengthy and thorough investigation, the source of almost half of these cases is eventually discovered. The Perkins family,

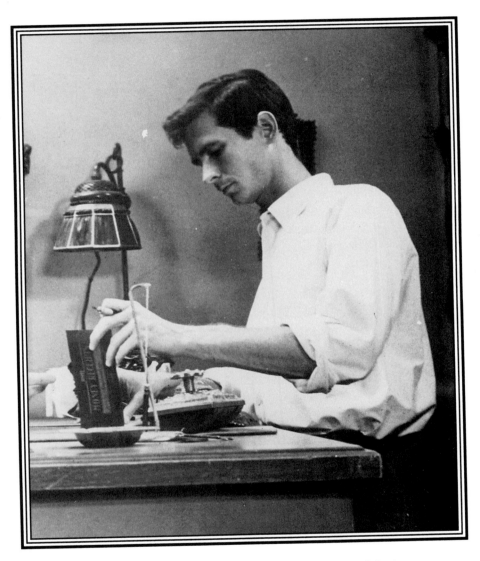

Anthony Perkins won wide acclaim for his portrayal of the insane motel manager, Norman Bates, in the 1960 thriller movie, *Psycho*.

however, had not yet identified how Perkins caught the disease.

Although infected with the deadly virus, Perkins was not ready to die. In 1983, he had said:

> It's satisfying to have grown from where I was to where I am. But there is so much growing still to be done. As long as I live, I'll be cleaning the past out of my mind, getting rid of those old cassettes I play over and over—my memories, my beliefs. I want to keep up with my life. Live it so completely that when death comes like a thief in the night, there'll be nothing left for him to steal.[8]

Perkins may have believed this now more than ever.

The family told very few people about the illness, hoping that most would have little faith in the tabloid story. Perkins felt that if anyone knew he was carrying the HIV virus, he would not get any more acting jobs. Still, he occasionally needed hospitalization. To maintain his privacy, he checked into the hospital using phony names.

Soon after learning of his HIV status, Perkins became involved in Project Angel Food, an organization that takes food to homebound people with AIDS. As volunteers, Perkins and his wife took meals to ill men, women, and children around Los Angeles. The actor's work with Project Angel Food was of immense personal significance. He once said that he learned "more about love, selflessness, and human understanding from the people I have met in this great adventure in the world of AIDS than I ever did in the cutthroat, competitive world in which I spent my life."[9]

Then Perkins became ill and bedridden. At times depression kept him from wanting to see anybody. When he did feel well enough to have visitors, friends came to share memories and tell him good-bye. At times Perkins told them he was ready to die. But according to Berenson, "he was just holding on, holding on for the boys and me."[10]

Berenson rarely left her husband's side during his last days. At night, she slept in a little bed next to his. During the day, she sometimes lay beside him to rest her head on his shoulder. She was with him when he died on September 12, 1992.

Anthony Perkins had traveled a great journey in his life, achieving a happiness for which he worked long and hard. He had built a successful career and a network of close friends. Most importantly to Perkins, he had built a happy family. No one would miss him as much as his wife and two sons. Standing next to him after he died, a grieving Berenson turned to a friend and asked, "Will it ever be the same without him?"[11]

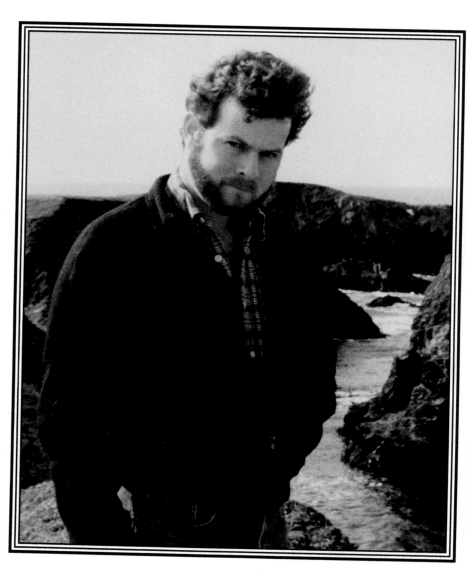

Randy Shilts

# Randy Shilts
## (1951–1994)

The doctor did not expect Randy Shilts to make it in 1993. He had been depressed after his emergency surgery and weakened by AIDS. Still, he held on. "When someone stood over me saying I was on the way out," Shilts later said, "it made my will to live kick in."[2] This will was driven by Shilts's determination to finish his third book, a ground-breaking work which would describe one of America's most sensitive social controversies.

Randy Shilts was born in 1951 in Davenport, Iowa. While he was young, his family lived in Aurora, Illinois, where his father sold prefabricated houses. His mother stayed home to care for Randy and his five brothers.

The Shilts family was religious and conservative.

Mr. Shilts belonged to a conservative political organization called the John Birch Society. It was not surprising, then, that when Randy himself became interested in politics, he started a local chapter of the Young Americans for Freedom, a John Birch Society youth group. Soon Randy was the club's state vice president. When he and the group had a falling out, Randy left and founded a local branch of the Students for a Democratic Society. This group's beliefs were more liberal and more in line with Randy's political philosophies.

After graduating from high school in 1969, Shilts spent one semester at nearby Aurora College. Then he transferred to Portland Community College in Portland, Oregon. After two years at the community college, Shilts enrolled in the University of Oregon in Eugene. He majored in English literature, but felt he lacked basic writing skills. Hoping to learn about grammar and punctuation, he took a journalism class. Shilts loved journalism—he had found his calling. Before long, he was the managing editor of the campus newspaper and was winning awards for his writing.

In Eugene, Shilts openly declared his homosexuality and became the head of Eugene's Gay People's Alliance. In his senior year of college, Shilts was elected the student body president. All of this extracurricular activity did not keep Shilts from his studies. He graduated at the head of his class in 1975 with a bachelor's degree in journalism.

After graduating, Shilts first worked as a correspondent for a gay magazine called *The Advocate*. Within the year he had moved to San Francisco to be a staff writer for the magazine. In addition, he was hired by a San Francisco television station to report on gay issues one day each week. In 1979, another television station hired Shilts to cover both city politics and gay issues.

In his work around San Francisco, Shilts became friends with various political leaders. One of them, Harvey Milk, was on the city's board of supervisors. Milk was gay and campaigned to eliminate discrimination against homosexuals. This was a volatile cause which many people vehemently opposed. One man, in fact, was so outraged by Milk's position on gay rights that he shot and killed both Milk and the mayor of San Francisco, George Moscone.

The murders shocked Shilts, who had begun writing a book about Milk's life. Shilts continued the biography, saying, "In doing the entire research on somebody else's life, you start to think about what life means. . . . I came away from [the project] truly inspired by the idea of how much one human being can accomplish."[3] *The Mayor of Castro Street: The Life and Times of Harvey Milk* was published in 1982 by St. Martin's Press. As a journalist, Shilts wanted to accomplish something, too. He made it his goal to write about topics that would not get written about otherwise.

He had his chance when he was hired as a

reporter for the *San Francisco Chronicle*. As such, Shilts became the first openly gay reporter for a major daily newspaper in America. The year was 1981 and the first cases of AIDS were just cropping up in San Francisco. Shilts found himself staring in the face of a story that would eventually rock the country. At that point, AIDS was just filtering into the nation's consciousness. Those who had even heard of the illness had little notion that it could infect them. Experts were calling the disease GRID, which stood for Gay-Related Immune Deficiency. Because of this and the publicity surrounding AIDS, many Americans believed it was an illness that attacked only gay men.

In fact, most media were not giving AIDS any coverage, but Shilts recognized AIDS as a major issue. He convinced the *Chronicle* to let him report on the disease full time, and became committed to alerting America about the disease. When he realized that his local reporting was having little effect on national awareness of AIDS, Shilts decided to write a book. At least fifteen publishers turned down his proposal before St. Martin's Press agreed to publish his book on the subject.

With sixteen thousand dollars in advance money, Shilts began his research. It did not take him long to spend all of the advance money in telephone calls and travel. But Shilts felt that his book was vitally important. AIDS was killing people he cared about and no one seemed to be paying attention.

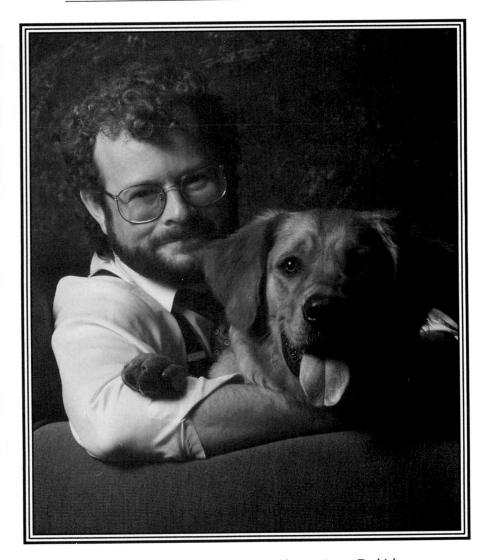

This photograph of Shilts with his golden retriever, Dashiel, was taken near the end of his life. Of the three books he wrote, *The Mayor Of Castro Street* was his favorite.

So once he spent the advance money, Shilts went into personal debt to finish the book.

In 1987, Shilts's book was published. *And the Band Played On: Politics, People, and the AIDS Epidemic* was a detailed examination of the first five years of AIDS in America. In the book, Shilts described how various groups grossly mismanaged the handling of the deadly disease. He criticized those who had ignored or covered up the scope and severity of AIDS for personal or political reasons. He accused the Reagan administration, the medical community, and even gay leaders of doing too little in response to the epidemic.[4]

The people Shilts criticized were angered by his book, but Shilts felt strongly that the truth was more important than the way people felt about him. He once commented, "Even though I hate [the criticism] I'm not going to adjust my writing so people don't yell at me. I've got to do what's right."[5]

Many agreed. Critics called Shilts's book "one of the most important books of the year" and an "impressive and pathbreaking piece of investigative journalism."[6] *And the Band Played On* was nominated for a National Book Award and remained on *The New York Times* best-seller list for five weeks. A television movie starring Richard Gere, Matthew Modine, and Anjelica Huston was made from the book and shown in 1993. It received high ratings and has been repeated several times since.

Having researched and written about AIDS since

its initial appearance, Shilts became aware of the danger of unprotected sex earlier than most people. While the rest of America was still trying to understand AIDS, Shilts was already practicing safe sex. Still, he had unknowingly put himself at risk prior to the first appearance of AIDS. Therefore, while working on *And the Band Played On*, he had himself tested for HIV. Because he did not want his personal situation to color his work, he told his doctor not to give him the test results until the book was completed. On the day Shilts turned in his finished manuscript, he learned he was HIV-positive.[7]

Shilts kept his HIV status a secret from the public. "To me it's no different than having high blood pressure or some other life-threatening illness," he said.[8] "Every gay writer who tests positive ends up being an AIDS activist. I wanted to keep on being a reporter."[9]

Shilts continued reporting while he lived in his San Francisco apartment or on his ten-acre ranch in the redwoods north of the city. Now he was a national correspondent for the *Chronicle*. He was also working on a new book, a book that would trace the history of homosexuals in the United States armed services.

For this work, Shilts interviewed gay people who were or had been in the military. He eventually talked to over a thousand people and verified their personal experiences with government records and documents. Shilts felt that the armed forces needlessly and cruelly discriminated against homosexuals. His book would be a collection of facts and real events that illustrated this. He said:

> I feel that prejudice in our society [against homosexuals] is born less out of malice than out of ignorance, and that if you just inform people . . . you can do more to erase prejudice than [you can by engaging in] any other kind of action.[10]

In his book, Shilts described the fear that gays in the armed forces live with. He recounted the military's methods of identifying homosexuals and how some officers rid their ranks of them. He even reported cases of beatings and suicides that were caused by hatred toward homosexuals.

Unfortunately, Shilts became seriously ill with AIDS before his book was finished. On Christmas Eve in 1992, one of his lungs collapsed. In January 1993, he underwent emergency surgery. In February of 1993, Shilts revealed to the public that he had AIDS. As he recovered from his operation, he became even more intent on completing his book. He wrote from his hospital bed. When he could not write, he dictated. His editor flew from New York to San Francisco to help him. Finally, the book was finished and *Conduct Unbecoming: Lesbians and Gays in the U.S. Military* was published in 1993. It, too, was a great success and soon hit the best-seller list. *The New York Times Book Review* called Shilts's third book "a sober, thoroughly researched and engrossingly readable history of the subject."[11] *Time* magazine called it a journalistic milestone.

Sadly, Shilts had little time to bask in the praise. Nor did he have the time to write any more books. On February 17, 1994, Randy Shilts, once acclaimed as "one of the outstanding journalists of our times,"[12] died of AIDS. He was only forty-two years old.

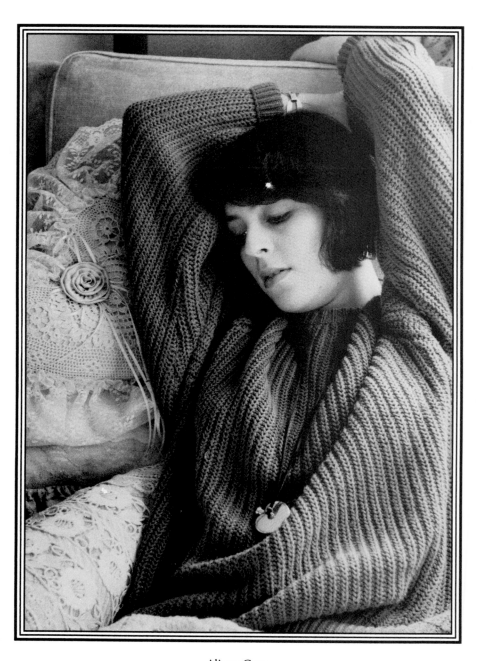

Alison Gertz

*There are times when you don't want to wake up in the morning, when you can't sleep, when you're angry life is so unfair, but the worst thing you can do is sit at home and think about the misery of your life. When you're given an opportunity to see how precious life is, it gives you an incentive to make the most of it. The only thing that matters is what we do with the time we have.*

—Alison Gertz[1]

# Alison Gertz
## (1966–1992)

"Baby, it's OK," Alison's mother whispered. "I love you. You're allowed to go."[2] Alison looked into her mother's eyes one last time and then she died.

When she had been well, Alison's quick smile had revealed her love of life. Just entering adulthood, she had hopes of marriage and dreams of children. She was an artistic young woman with a promising career ahead of her. Now, none of her dreams would come true. Alison was dead, her future ripped from her by a disease that killed everything in its path. Twenty-six-year-old Alison Gertz had been stolen by AIDS.

Alison was born on February 27, 1966. Her father, Jerrold Gertz, was a real-estate investor. Carol, her mother, operated a national chain of fashion stores. The Gertzes lived on Park Avenue in New York City, in an atmosphere of affluence and social prominence. They were able to give their only child opportunities most parents could not. The Gertzes sent Alison to private school, and in the summers, the family vacationed at Westhampton Beach on Long Island. There, Alison loved to sail about the bay in her own little boat called the *Ali Cat*.

As a teenager, Alison was no wallflower. She liked to laugh and have fun, and always wanted to be in the middle of the action.

She was a pretty girl and had many friends. Together, they enjoyed various New York City night spots. At one, Studio 54, Alison met a handsome bartender with whom she became good friends. Alison once described him as "the most beautiful man I'd ever seen. We were like brother and sister for a year, except that there was a very strong physical attraction."[3]

When Alison's parents left town for a weekend in the summer of 1982, she invited the man over to her family's apartment. He came bringing champagne and roses, and, although neither one knew it then, he also brought AIDS.[4]

That night they had sexual intercourse—once. Although Alison had protected herself against pregnancy, the man had not used a condom. The night was not the romantic beginning to a love affair. There had been no sparks, and it was clear to both Alison and her friend that there would be no lasting relationship. The night had been significant, however; it was the night Alison began to die. She was sixteen.

At the time, Alison had no idea the HIV virus had entered her body and was waiting in deadly ambush. AIDS was a new disease then, and neither Alison nor the general public knew how dangerous unprotected sex could be. So Alison carried on with her life in much the same way as other teens did.

Alison graduated with honors from high school and entered Parsons School of Design, an art college in New York City. After completing her junior year there, she felt ready to pursue a career in art and signed on with an agent who would help her find work as a freelance illustrator.

Alison's personal life was full, too. She had three very best friends—Dini, Victoria, and Stefani—with whom she went to parties and talked about life. She had a boyfriend she had been seeing for three years. During this time, she had occasional bouts with fevers and diarrhea, but because none lasted long, Alison and her parents believed her brief illnesses were episodes of the flu.

In 1988, Alison came down with a fever she could not shake. Alison's mother insisted she check into the hospital to find out the cause. Over a two-week period, the doctors tested Alison for everything they could think of, but could find nothing wrong with her. No one considered testing Alison for AIDS. At the time, AIDS was thought to be a disease that struck only gay men, people who had received blood transfusions, or intravenous drug users. Alison was none of these.

Then a doctor noticed something strange on Alison's lung X-ray. After performing a biopsy, he diagnosed her as having PCP, a rare type of pneumonia now often seen in AIDS patients. Alison's doctor was shocked and saddened to realize that Alison had AIDS.[5] He gave her the news with tears in his eyes.

Where had Alison's infection come from? To her relief, her boyfriend checked negative for HIV. Then, on a hunch, she started looking for her bartender friend from Studio 54—and learned that he had died of AIDS.[6] It was then that Alison knew how she had been infected.

Alison's first reaction to her diagnosis was panic and fear. She did not want to die. The news tore her parents apart, but they stayed outwardly strong for their daughter's sake.

After the initial shock, Alison began reading about people who had lived with AIDS for more than eight years. This gave her hope and she decided that being depressed was a huge waste of energy. She came to view AIDS as a challenge and felt she must turn her illness into something positive. "I want to help other people," Alison said. "I want to believe that there is some purpose to my being sick."[7]

When Alison's mother read a series of articles in *The New York Times* about AIDS, she noticed that it did not address heterosexual transmission of the disease. Feeling that this was an alarming omission, she suggested that Alison share her experience with the newspaper. Alison was enthusiastic. In 1989, Alison's story, one of the first about middle-class heterosexual AIDS, hit the newsstands. Soon it was retold by newspapers all over the world. In addition, the World Health Organization made a film about Alison which was shown at the United Nations on World AIDS Day in 1989. Since then, the movie has traveled to many countries. Alison's selfless sharing of her private tragedy led *Esquire* magazine to name her its 1989 "Woman of the Year."

In the meantime, Alison's parents organized a group called Concerned Parents for AIDS Research. It is still active and has raised nearly $2 million for research on finding a cure for AIDS. Mr. and Mrs. Gertz never stopped hoping a cure would come in time to save their daughter. In addition, they were determined to increase America's awareness of the disease. According to Mrs. Gertz, "We never hid [Alison's illness]. So many parents refuse to believe that their children are sexually active and can contract this disease. We can't put our heads in the sand and say it's not happening."[8]

In a very short time, Alison became a symbol of how anybody could be infected with HIV. As a pioneer in educating middle-class heterosexuals about AIDS, Alison was a guest on many nationwide television programs including "Oprah Winfrey," "20/20," "Good Morning America," and "Sally Jessy

Raphael." Alison's purpose in appearing was to educate teenagers. She believed that the best education for young people came from young people. She said, "They might not listen to their parents or pay attention to the news, but they might understand it coming from me because I'm one of them."[9] So, as often as possible, she spoke to high school and college students. During these visits, Alison tried to impress upon her audiences the urgency of her message. Young people, she told them, were the second-fastest growing group of HIV-infected people in America.

In 1992, actress Molly Ringwald portrayed Alison in a television movie called *Something to Live For, The Alison Gertz Story*. During the twenty-four hours after it was broadcast, nearly one hundred ninety thousand people called the National AIDS Hotline with questions about the disease. This set a record and prompted the U.S. Department of Health and Human Services to present Alison with an award for exceptional public service.

That same year Alison became very sick. Lying next to a bedside table full of pills, she said:

> I hope in the next few years there will be a cure . . . there are so many things I want to accomplish. I want to get back to my painting. I'd like to do some traveling. . . . I think I'd be an excellent mother. I'd like to live in a house in the country and have a million cats and lots of dogs.[10]

Alison knew these were dreams. The truth was

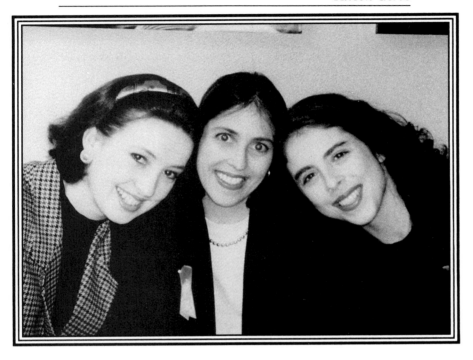

Victoria Leacock (left) and Dini von Mueffling (right) wait with Alison Gertz (center) for a 1992 appearance on the "Sally Jessy Raphael" show.

that she might not live much longer. Courageously facing death, she pledged to be as happy as she could with whatever time she had left. Alison's parents and friends helped her to achieve that goal. Her mother spent most of her time at Alison's apartment, and her father came every morning to walk her dog and make Alison breakfast. Dini, Victoria, and Stefani were also close by and helped care for their ailing friend.

Alison had always been a spiritual person and had studied many different religions. She became even more spiritual once she fell ill with AIDS. Her belief in a life after death, along with the love and support of her family and friends, were a great source of strength. Therefore, she was never afraid of dying.

Unfortunately, all the love in the world could not cure AIDS. Alison suffered through night sweats, chills, fevers, and pain. Her once healthy five-foot-eight-inch frame dropped to 112 pounds, and though she had fought it gallantly, Alison could no longer keep death from her door.

On August 8, 1992, Alison Gertz died of AIDS at her family's summer home in Westhampton Beach.[11] Alison's body was cremated. Then, one beautiful evening, her parents and doctor took a boat into the bay where Alison had spent so many happy hours. As the sun set, they scattered Alison's ashes.

Alison was not really gone. She lived on through her three loyal friends who firmly established the AIDS awareness organization Alison had envisioned creating. Now Dini von Mueffling, Victoria Leacock, and Stefani Greenfield administer the foundation called Love Heals. They take Alison's message to America's young people, speaking only where adults will let them talk uncensored. They tell youth that women are the fastest growing group of people being infected with HIV and that teenagers are the second fastest growing group. They also tell them that 70 percent of all new HIV infections in the United States are through heterosexual sex, but that only 10 percent of HIV-infected teenagers know they are carrying the virus.

For their presentations, the women show a twenty-minute documentary about Alison which was filmed by Leacock. Not all of the scenes show Alison looking beautiful. "Ali was gorgeous," Greenfield said, "but people have to see the beginning, middle, and end."[12]

After one school visit, counselors told von Mueffling, Leacock, and Greenfield that even they had learned things about AIDS. One girl privately told them how her own friend had died of AIDS, though she had been told that the friend had cancer. The girl then handed them one hundred dollars as a contribution to Love Heals. In this same way, von Mueffling said, she and her friends had been moved to action by Alison's life and death.

To the world, Alison had become a symbol that anyone can be at risk of catching AIDS, but Alison was not a symbol to her friends. According to von Mueffling:

> She was our best friend—the one we went dancing with, went to the movies with, the one we cried over bad boyfriends with. Then suddenly Ali became the one we went to Oprah with, on speaking engagements with, and to the hospital to visit. Later, she became the one whose diaper we changed. . . . The three of us cannot be silent. Ali cannot have worked so hard and died for nothing.[13]

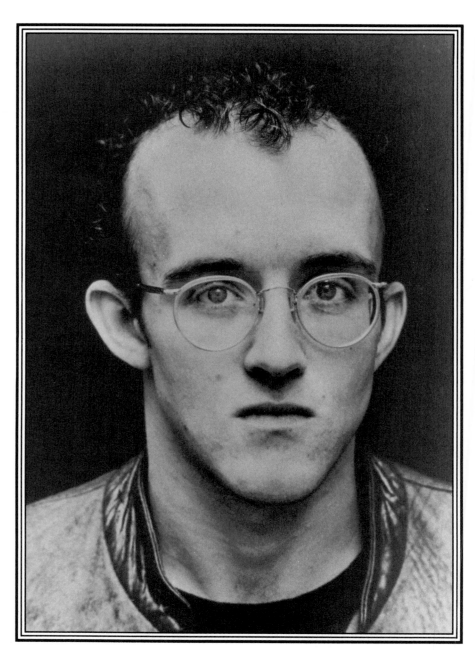

Keith Haring

*He was one of the most astonishingly unique talents of recent times.*

—Tony Shafrazi[1]

# Keith Haring
## (1958–1990)

The New York City police officer handcuffed the young man and led him to the station. The criminal had been caught red-handed, so there was no point in his denying his guilt. What was the man's crime? Was he a thief, or a murderer? Actually, the police had arrested an artist while he was creating art. Unfortunately, he was doing it without permission on public walls, an act that is illegal in New York, as in most cities. The man was not a common vandal. He was Keith Haring, a highly respected artist who deeply believed in taking his art to the streets.

Keith Haring was born on May 4, 1958, in Kutztown, Pennsylvania. As a young boy, he had a lively imagination and liked to make up wild and funny stories. Television shows like "My Favorite Martian" fueled his fantasies and he often illustrated his tales. Keith's father liked to draw, too, and encouraged his son's art. Keith's developing style was cartoonlike, influenced by "The Flintstones" and "The Jetsons." If anyone had asked Keith what he wanted to be when he grew up, he would have said Walt Disney or Dr. Seuss.

Keith attended school in Kutztown, but sensed that he belonged among artists. Within a year of his high school graduation, he was living in New York City, a mecca for artists of all kinds.

In 1979, Haring enrolled in Manhattan's School of Visual Arts. There he sketched on great lengths of paper that he rolled across the floor, out the door, and onto the city sidewalk. People walking by would stop to watch him work and talk about his art. "Most of them weren't the type that go to art galleries," Haring later said, "but a lot of their comments struck me as more perceptive than those of my teachers and fellow students."[2] After a year at the art school, Haring was ready to move on. Ever since his arrival in New York, he had been intrigued by an unlikely source of art—the graffiti he saw in subway stations. Some of the work was tasteless vandalism and some was meaningless, but Haring found much of the art more exciting than what he saw in New York City museums. He viewed the subway system as an art gallery for the city's thousands of commuters.

Inspired, Haring became a graffiti artist himself.

Not wanting to deface public property, he confined his artwork to billboards which were not being used. These were covered with black paper by city authorities. Even so, drawing or writing on them was against the law and Haring had to work at lightning speed to avoid police.

Haring used white chalk drawings on black billboards as his new sketchpad. The more he drew, the more a unique style emerged. Haring most liked making cookie cutter-type outlines of objects such as crawling babies and alligator-jawed dogs. It was not long before his distinctive style became familiar to New York City's commuters, though few knew his name nor would they recognize him if they saw him.

But people in the art world were learning Haring's name. When he moved to New York, he had found an apartment in a downtown neighborhood where many young artists lived. Because the artists frequented the same cafes, coffee houses, and dance clubs, they became acquainted with one another. Often, they would decorate the walls of the neighborhood hangouts or display their artwork there. In this way, they became familiar with each other's work. Haring, too, showed his work around the neighborhood, and it was not long before he became known and his style recognized.

After art gallery owner Tony Shafrazi gave Haring a solo exhibit in 1981, his career exploded. Over the next three years Haring's work was exhibited in a dizzying array of places around the world, including the cities of Pittsburgh, San Francisco, Washington, D.C., London, São Paulo, and Venice. In 1984, a book called *Art in Transit* was made from photographs of Haring's subway drawings. Haring's work could also be seen in less conventional settings: a set for an MTV program, discotheque walls, the sides of school buildings, even a billboard at New York's Times Square.

All the while, Haring was growing as an artist. Now he was being influenced by pop artist Andy Warhol, and elements from primitive Aztec and African art were making their way into his work. Haring was also busy studying a science called semiotics, the study of signs and symbols, and original hieroglyphics began showing up in his art work. Little by little, Haring was developing a "vocabulary," a set of pictograms he used in various pieces of art.

This vocabulary seemed able to communicate with people everywhere. In 1985, Haring was invited to France to make a mural illustrating the Bible's Ten Commandments. In 1986, a West German museum invited Haring to paint a mural on the Berlin Wall. When he arrived in West Germany, Haring was surprised to find that gun-toting East German guards actually patrolled both sides of the Wall. This frightened Haring who said, "I have never dealt with the fear of being shot."[3] However, his work proceeded and when he finished, he had created a hundred-yard-long chain of interlocked human beings. The colors he used—red, black, and yellow—were the colors of the West and East German flags. Haring hoped his art would express the senselessness of "walls and enemies and borders" and he wanted his painting to psychologically destroy the Wall.[4]

By now, Haring was also working with sculpture, and painting in oils and acrylics. His popularity had soared and along with it, the prices people were paying for his work. Eventually, he would mount forty-two one-man exhibitions. In 1985, the *Washington Post* called him "the hottest artist in New York at the moment."[5]

Although the recognition was gratifying, Haring still found himself drawing in subway stations from time to time. He liked being accessible to everyday people and was committed to sharing his art in places other than galleries and museums. Of this work, Haring said, "the stuff I do in the subways is still every bit as important to me as the work I show in galleries. I give it just as much thought as a painting that I sell for 10 or 20 thousand dollars."[6] This belief ran so deep that Haring was willing to risk being arrested—between 1984 and 1986, he was arrested five times. Sometimes, he was taken to the police station, ticketed, then released—and asked for his autograph.

In fact, Haring was becoming as much of a celebrity as the people he was seen with—among them Andy Warhol, Yoko Ono, Madonna, and Brooke Shields. Just as often, though, Haring spent time with lesser-known people. He liked to visit elementary

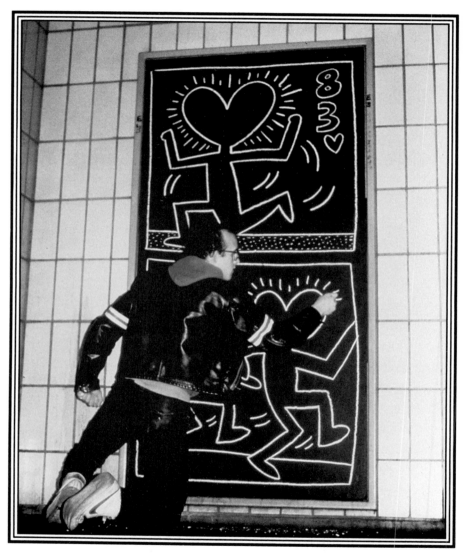

Keith Haring's white chalk drawings like these became a familiar site to New York City's subway commuters during the 1980s.

schools and would graciously sign autographs upon request. When he invited three thousand guests to his birthday parties, the street kids there usually outnumbered the stars. To many of the young people Haring was a sincere friend, and one youth described him as "a cool dude to hang out with."[7] Art historian Henry Geldzahler saw more to Haring than this. "He's gentle in person," he said, "but his character is *very* directed."[8]

To spread his art more widely, Haring opened a store in New York in 1986 called the Pop Shop. There he sold T-shirts, jeans, watches, buttons, refrigerator magnets, and coloring books all emblazoned with his "vocabulary." Some people criticized Haring's new venture, saying one could not mass-produce art. To these critics, he replied, "You don't communicate the same way you did twenty years ago, or fifty. You can't just stay in your studio and paint; that's not the most effective way to communicate."[9]

As time passed, Haring's work began promoting social causes. He created artwork in support of the antiapartheid movement, nuclear disarmament, and famine relief. Increasingly, he wanted to communicate significant ideas to the world. He drew faceless people being zapped by flying saucers, monsters with computers as heads, and humans being fed into machines. Haring seemed to be warning society of the dangers of too much technology.

This work warned of other dangers as well.

In one painting, his usually playful figures were suffering, surrounded by skulls with wings. Many people thought this piece was about AIDS, an illness of great personal significance to Haring.

Since moving to New York City, Haring had been open about his homosexuality. He had practiced safe sex during most of these years, but felt he had probably been exposed to the HIV virus before its existence was known. Therefore, when Haring learned he was HIV-positive, he was not surprised.

During the late 1980s, Haring watched AIDS kill more and more of his friends. This moved him to action. He created AIDS-related art to sell at the Pop Shop. He also worked to educate young people about HIV infection and often passed out safe sex stickers, believing, as he said, that "when people are treated as if they have some intelligence and are given explicit information, they appreciate it. And it's the only thing that gets through to kids, the people that need it."[10]

Haring even joined ACT UP, an organization that staged demonstrations to call the public's attention to AIDS. Many of ACT UP's tactics were controversial and some critics found their methods offensive. To them, ACT UP spokesperson Larry Kramer replied, "We're not here to make friends, we're here to raise issues."[11] Haring believed that openness about these issues was essential.

To Haring, one of the hardest parts of facing his own AIDS illness was "knowing that there's so much more stuff to do. I'm a complete workaholic. I'm so scared that one day I'll wake up and I won't be able to do it."[12] Even if there were five of him, Haring said, there would be too much to do. Yet he felt comfort in knowing he had lived life doing what he wanted. His art expressed his feelings and made people think. Unfortunately, he never had the chance to share all of his ideas.

On February 16, 1990, Keith Haring died of AIDS.[13] He was thirty-one years old. His loss can never be measured, for who knows what the artwork he might have created could have taught us about ourselves?

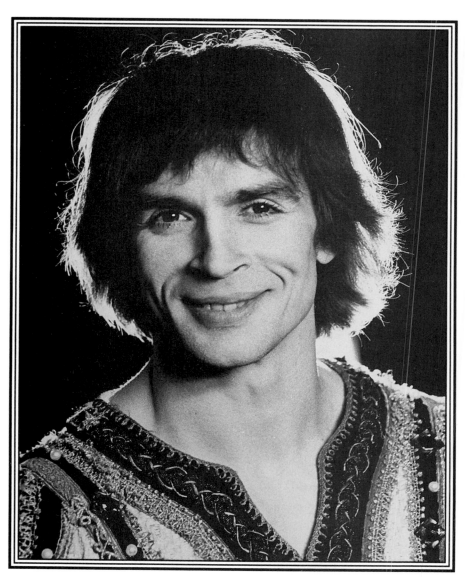

Rudolf Nureyev

*What he wanted was simply to dance, every night, everywhere.*

—Mikhail Baryshnikov[1]

# Rudolf Nureyev
## (1938–1993)

The Royal Ballet's audience sat spellbound in the darkened theater. Since he defected from the Kirov Ballet, there had been rumors that Rudolf Nureyev's powers as a dancer were unequaled. Now, as fans watched him partner the company's prima ballerina, Margot Fonteyn, they were not disappointed. England's most famous ballerina seemed inspired to fresh heights by the young Russian's passionate, almost electric energy; his great leaps seemed to hold him suspended in the air. When the ballet ended, the audience exploded in cheers. Fonteyn plucked a rose from the masses of flowers being thrown on stage and held it tenderly to her lips. Then she offered it to the Russian. Taking the rose, he dropped immediately to one knee and kissed Fonteyn's hand.

Again, the audience thundered applause. It was 1962 and Rudolf Nureyev was about to set the Western dance world on fire.

Rudolf was born in 1938 on a train speeding across southern Siberia. His mother was on her way to Vladivostok where his father was stationed in the Soviet army. Rudolf's father was transferred to Moscow next; his family followed. In 1941, Mr. Nureyev left to fight in World War II. Soon German bombs forced Mrs. Nureyev and her children to leave Moscow. They eventually settled in Ufa, a remote town at the foot of the Ural Mountains.

Poverty forced the Nureyevs to share a one-room house with four other people. There they lived almost entirely on potatoes, but even this meager food was scarce. Once Rudolf's mother walked almost forty miles to find food for her children's supper. Rudolf would never forget the "consistent, gnawing hunger" of his early years.[2]

Yet young Rudolf's life was not without pleasure. He liked being alone and often climbed to the top of a hill to watch Ufa's townspeople go about their business. He was mesmerized by the music on his family's radio. At seven, he was learning folk dancing at school, and at home he sang and danced until bedtime. When people saw him dance, they would tell his mother, "Rudi's got a natural talent for dancing. . . . It's a gift . . . you ought to send him to the Leningrad Ballet School."[3]

The Leningrad Ballet School—the very sound of

it thrilled Rudolf, though he had little idea of what ballet was. He was sure of one thing though—if it had to do with dancing, it was where he wanted to be.

Rudolf saw his first ballet when he was seven years old. The moment he entered the theater, he was transported beyond Ufa to a place of his dreams. Years later, Rudolf remembered the theater's "soft beautiful lights and gleaming crystal chandeliers . . . everywhere velvet . . . gold—another world, a place which, to my dazzled eyes, you could only hope to encounter in the most enchanted fairy tale."[4]

When the dancing began, Rudolf was caught in a spell from which he would never emerge. Now a new hunger filled him, for he knew he had been born to dance. Although there were no proper ballet schools in Ufa, he found people who taught him some ballet. As he practiced, the refrain, "To Leningrad, to Leningrad" echoed in his head.

But how? The Nureyevs' finances made Rudolf's dream impossible. Furthermore, his father was now home from the war and strongly opposed to Rudolf's dancing. He wanted his son to get a good education, but Rudolf had no interest in school. On one report card, a teacher remarked, "[Rudolf] jumps like a frog and that's about all he knows. He even dances on the staircase landings."[5]

In desperation, Mr. Nureyev forbade Rudolf to dance. Still, Rudolf would not stop. He lied to get out of the house to take ballet lessons, and by the time he was sixteen, he was secretly performing small roles in Ufa ballets. When Rudolf began earning money for his dancing, his father reluctantly accepted his son's chosen career.

By now Rudolf knew all about the Soviet Union's most famous dance school, Leningrad's Kirov Ballet. With high hopes, he bought himself a one-way ticket to Leningrad.

At the age of seventeen, Rudolf was woefully behind in the technical training most dancers already had. His desire, however, overflowed. Stepping forward to audition for the Kirov School, Rudolf danced with all his heart. When he finished, one teacher remarked, "Young man, you'll become either a brilliant dancer or a total failure—and most likely you'll be a failure!"[6]

Like this teacher, other Kirov instructors noted something unusual about Rudolf's dancing—an unconcealed jubilance that many of the perfectly trained dancers lacked. Hoping to harness this natural joy with classical Russian technique, the Kirov accepted Rudolf.

Finally enrolled at a proper ballet school, Nureyev practiced relentlessly, wanting to make up for lost years. Often he worked alone in the dance studio after everyone else had gone home. Three years after entering the Kirov School, Nureyev earned a position in its dance company, the Kirov Dance Company. His dance roles grew steadily in number and importance until he was dancing the lead male parts in classic ballets such as *Giselle* and *Swan Lake*.

Although Nureyev's dancing was heralded, he was winning no popularity contests with the people at the Kirov. First, he refused to join a Communist club. He had no interest in politics; all he cared about was dancing. By not joining, Nureyev was rejecting the Communist party and, therefore, the Soviet government. This jeopardized the standing of the Kirov Ballet Company, which depended on the government's support. Nureyev's attitude angered many people there.

To make matters worse, Nureyev was rebellious in other ways: He went out at night when he was not supposed to and ignored curfews. In spite of warnings not to mix with foreigners, Nureyev would talk with foreign dancers during their rare appearances in Leningrad. Over and over again, Nureyev drew disapproval from the Kirov.

He was somewhat surprised, therefore, to learn he had been selected to accompany the Kirov on its 1961 tour of Paris and London. In Paris, Nureyev's dancing was spectacular. Between performances, he characteristically defied instructions and toured the city with his new foreign friends.

On the day the Kirov dancers gathered at the airport to fly to London, Nureyev was pulled aside. Plans for him had been changed, the director said. He would not be going to London, but flying home to perform at the Kremlin. Nureyev was not fooled. He knew he was being sent back to the Soviet Union as a punishment for his behavior.

Nureyev realized his moment had come. If he did not act now, he might never leave the Soviet Union again. This thought horrified him—and it gave him courage. He slipped away from the dancers and threw himself at two French policemen, saying he wanted to stay in Paris. French officials placed Nureyev in protective custody and would not release him to the Soviet officials who asked for his return. Nureyev had defected.

Less than one week after his defection, Nureyev was back on stage, now dancing with a French ballet company. Then, in 1962, England's famous ballerina, Dame Margot Fonteyn, asked him to dance with her. Their debut for London's Royal Ballet Company was a sensation that marked the beginning of a long partnership.

For the next two decades, Nureyev ignited audiences all over the world. Maintaining his independence, he never joined any one dance company. Instead, he worked as a guest artist with various troupes, coming and going at will.

Wherever he danced, people swooned. Normally quiet, dignified ballet audiences screamed when Nureyev leaped. People who had never been to the ballet before became fans. Perhaps critic Laura Shapiro captured Nureyev's essence best when she wrote, "The raw vigor of his flamboyant leaps, the animal rapture that propelled him in huge turns around the stage, the passion that smoldered as he bent over his partner—it was all excess, and it was all gorgeous."[7]

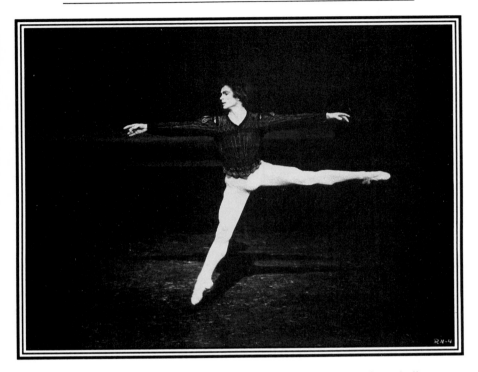

After defecting from the Soviet Union, Rudolf Nureyev danced all over the world. This performance of *Swan Lake* is with the American Ballet Theatre.

Always growing, always expanding, Nureyev seemed constantly in motion. When he was not dancing, he was choreographing. He brought Russian ballets to the western world, and reworked classic ballets. He created his own dances and experimented with modern dance. By 1980, he had danced with a multitude of major companies including troupes in America, Australia, Argentina, Germany, Canada, and Switzerland.

Nureyev's life outside ballet was also in constant

motion. He traveled incessantly and owned homes in New York, France, and Italy. Between ballets and jetting here and there, Nureyev visited art galleries and museums, and listened to music. Whenever possible, he would watch other people perform, drinking in the arts like a man dying of thirst.

Nureyev had a reputation for being unconventional and living life in the fast lane. In his early twenties, he fell in love with the Danish ballet dancer Erik Bruhn, and made no secret of their relationship. Throughout the 1970s and 1980s, Nureyev frequented nightclubs and parties, often in the company of famous people. Yet he was always guarded about his private life, believing that the public did not have the right to know everything about him.

Nureyev was also guarded about the illness that would eventually take his life. It was not until his death that most people learned he had been HIV-positive for many years.[8] Keeping his illness a secret, Nureyev remained on stage for as long as possible. As he neared his fiftieth birthday, his dancing was not as strong as it had been in his youth and many critics suggested that it was time for him to retire. His reply was, "Inside I am only twenty-three, an eternal youth. Dancing, for me, is forever."[9]

In 1991, Nureyev became seriously ill, but still he would not stop. He had created a new choreography for a classic ballet, *La Bayadère* for the Paris Opera Ballet, and he was determined to see the project through. During the 1992 rehearsals, he left his hospital bed to oversee the production's progress. When the ballet premiered in October, Nureyev was there.

As two dancers helped him to stand on stage, the audience honored Nureyev with an ovation that lasted a full ten minutes. Flowers showered down on him as ballet fans thanked the man who had touched them with his joy of dance.

Rudolf Nureyev died on January 6, 1993. Although his doctor reported that he died of "a cardiac complication following a grievous illness," most people believed his death came from complications due to AIDS.[10] He was fifty-four years old.

Of his friend, fellow dancer Mikhail Baryshnikov said:

> He was an amazingly beautiful dancer, but what made him so irreplaceable was the *generosity* of his dancing—his joy in his talent, the power of his fantasy, and his sharing it all with you. There he was, exploding, and you couldn't not watch him. No matter what he was doing, he was always at the same time, giving you this message: "Stay with me. Watch. It's something wonderful. Wait till I show you."[11]

Indeed, it had been something wonderful.

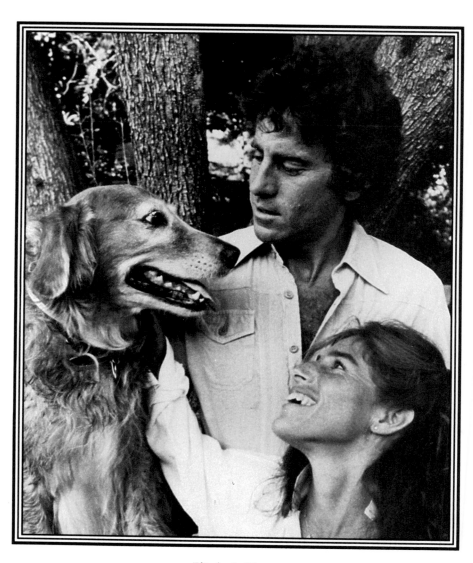

Elizabeth Glaser

*It was [my daughter] who taught me to love when all I wanted to do was hate. She taught me to be brave when all I felt was fear. And she taught me to help others when all I wanted to do was help myself.*

—Elizabeth Glaser[1]

# Elizabeth Glaser
## (1947–1994)

When the doctors told Elizabeth Glaser that her beautiful little girl was dying from AIDS, it was more pain than she could bear. "A mother's job," she said, "is to save her child; it's a basic animal instinct. But I was failing. I had to do more."[2] In those terrible moments Glaser vowed to become active in the fight against the disease, and she spent the last years of her life doing just that.

Elizabeth Ann Meyer was born in New York in 1947. She grew up in the suburbs of Long Island where her father was a successful businessman. Mrs. Meyer, Elizabeth's mother, was a

67

director of urban renewal projects that built homes for the poor. From her mother's example, Elizabeth learned it was her responsibility to help people less fortunate than she. After high school, Elizabeth attended Boston University and earned a master's degree in education. When her first marriage ended in divorce, she moved to Los Angeles to teach elementary school. She also worked as a director of the Los Angeles Children's Museum.

Elizabeth met Paul Michael Glaser when she was twenty-seven years old, and it was love at first sight. As the star of a new television show, "Starsky and Hutch," Paul became an overnight success. During the four years the show was popular, he was recognized everywhere he went. However, he and Elizabeth, who were now constant companions, stayed out of the Hollywood spotlight. Instead, they spent their free time with close friends.

Elizabeth and Paul were married in 1980. In 1981, their first child, Ariel, was born. Shortly after the delivery, Elizabeth began hemorrhaging (losing blood rapidly and uncontrollably). As she watched, doctors pumped transfusions into her, unaware that a deadly HIV virus was lurking inside the life-saving blood.[3] While Elizabeth recovered from the birth and breast-fed her daughter, no one suspected she had been infected with HIV. It would be years before the virus was discovered. In the meantime, tragically, Elizabeth transferred it to Ariel through her breast milk.

For now, though, the Glasers' lives were blissful. Elizabeth and Ariel were healthy, and Paul's acting career was successful. In time he would become an accomplished movie director. The Glasers bought a big house in Santa Monica, California, where they planned to raise several happy, romping children.

When Elizabeth became pregnant for a second time, she still did not know that she was carrying HIV. In the womb, she passed the virus on again to her unborn child. In 1984, the Glasers' son, Jacob (Jake), was born. He, too, seemed healthy, and the Glasers' lives proceeded in fairy-tale-like progression, but their storybook existence was near an end.

About a year after Jake's birth, Ariel began having stomach pains and fatigue. No one could explain why she had these problems. Finally, doctors discovered that she had AIDS.[4] The Glasers were devastated. At first, Elizabeth could barely contain her grief and anger. Sometimes she would climb into her car and scream at God, "I hate you for letting Ari get sick! I hate you for making this my life!"[5] When the rest of the family was tested for the HIV virus, Elizabeth learned that the nightmare had only just begun. Although Paul had escaped infection, both Jake and Elizabeth were HIV-positive.[6] At times, this was more than Elizabeth could bear, and she sometimes thought about committing suicide.

Slowly, though, she realized that if she gave up, she eliminated the possibility of being able to benefit should a cure come along.

So Elizabeth tried to live life as normally as possible. Because the Glasers had heard of the ostracism, rejection, and hatred other AIDS victims had suffered, they kept their illnesses a secret. They did share the information with a few friends whom they swore to secrecy. At this time, little was known about how AIDS was transferred from one person to another, so the Glasers lived in isolation for almost a year. "I cried every night," Elizabeth later said, "and I kept wishing for things that never seemed to happen. I wished that Ari would be invited for a sleep-over, that Jake would be invited for a play date, that Paul and I would be invited to a dinner party."[7]

When the U.S. Surgeon General announced that AIDS could not be transmitted through casual contact, the Glasers began socializing again. Even so, seeing other people with normal lives and healthy children was difficult for Elizabeth. Often, she wished for an angel to appear and take her family's illnesses away, but there were no angels.

Gradually, Elizabeth realized that little was known about AIDS in children because few people were researching pediatric AIDS. AZT, a drug which had proven effective in combatting AIDS in adults, was not yet available for youngsters. Through

Elizabeth's persistence, Ariel became one of the first children in the country to be treated with AZT. In her fight to secure the drug for her daughter, Elizabeth said she had felt like a pioneer in the first wagon train West.

During the summer of 1987, despite the AZT treatments, Ariel became seriously ill. Throughout the fall and winter she grew weak and thin, and suffered frequent pain. By February, she could not walk or talk. Elizabeth carried her daughter everywhere and took her for walks in a stroller. The spring and summer brought no relief, and Ariel was hospitalized in August. There was nothing the doctors could do. Shortly after Ariel's seventh birthday, she died.

Her daughter's death spurred Elizabeth to action. She worried about Jake and was determined to do whatever she could to try to save him. To do so, Elizabeth knew she must get scientists to study AIDS in children. She traveled to Washington, D.C., to convince policymakers to allocate more money to pediatric AIDS research. She met with the President and members of Congress. She gave speeches and appeared on national television. Wherever she went and whomever she spoke to, her message was straightforward and forceful. "Every person with AIDS is somebody's child," she would say. "AIDS is not a political issue. It's a virus and it kills people, no matter who they are."[8] Elizabeth stressed the urgency of her fight, and saw herself as an advocate for

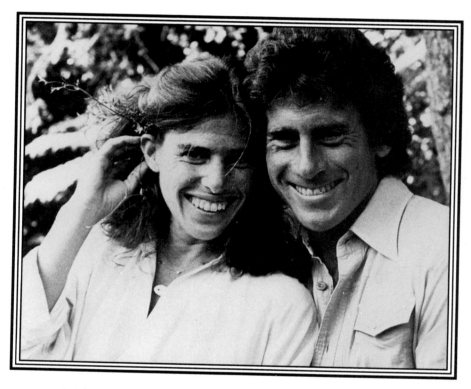

As Elizabeth waged her public fight against AIDS, Paul stayed in the background, offering his quiet support.

the thousands of children with AIDS who could not fight for themselves.

Yet for Elizabeth, too, the clock was ticking and her lobbying efforts were taking too long. So, in 1988, she and two friends founded the Pediatric AIDS Foundation (PAF), an organization created to raise money for research on AIDS in children.

To call further attention to the plight of those with AIDS, Elizabeth and author Laura Palmer wrote a book recounting her family's private tragedy. *In the Absence of Angels* (1991) was praised as courageous, heroic, and extraordinary. Always seeking opportunities to take the AIDS issue to the public, Elizabeth spoke at the 1992 Democratic National Convention. Her speech of profound sadness and frustration riveted a national audience.

> When you cry for help and no one listens, you start to lose your hope. I began to lose faith in America. I felt my country was letting me down, and it was. This is not the America I was raised to be proud of. I was raised to believe that others' problems were my problems as well.[9]

When Elizabeth's problems overwhelmed her, she said, she thought about Ariel. "I am active in fighting AIDS because I want to be a person [Ariel] would be proud of; I was so proud of her. And Ari is always with me. In my weaker moments, I think about her courage and I am able to go on."[10]

During her last years, Elizabeth worked tirelessly at PAF, which has raised over $30 million for pediatric AIDS research. In addition, she urged ordinary people to become heroes in the battle against AIDS. "It may simply mean breaking the polite silence that follows when someone makes an ignorant or intolerant remark about people with AIDS. If you take a stand with that one person, you take a stand for millions of families like mine."[11]

Although she was busy, Elizabeth was careful to reserve time for life's everyday, simple joys. This included generous portions of attention to Jake, who had grown into an active boy who loved ball games and bike riding.

In August 1994, Elizabeth's health deteriorated. More and more of her days were spent watching Jake from a bedroom window while he played in the yard. As her condition worsened, she clung to the hope that an AIDS cure would be found in time to save her son. By December, Elizabeth could no longer speak. On the third day of the month, she died.

Elizabeth's friend Bob Hattoy, said of her: "[She] taught me that it's not the length of our lives, it's the depth. It's not about dying with AIDS, it's about living with AIDS. She rose to the challenge."[12]

According to her wishes, Elizabeth was buried

next to Ariel. As he grieved for his wife, Paul Glaser noted that Elizabeth's work had been left unfinished. He hoped that her death would inspire America to increase its efforts to conquer AIDS. Only then would Elizabeth's dream for all of the "Jakes" of the world be fulfilled.

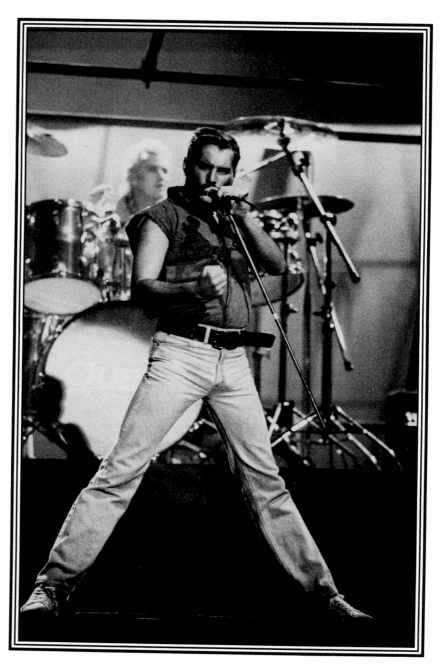

Freddie Mercury

# Freddie Mercury
## (1946–1991)

Some people say there is a quality that a few people are born with that sets them apart from the rest of the world. This quality often appears at an early age and is what makes them stars—stars like rock musician Freddie Mercury, who with his band, Queen, recorded eighteen albums which sold more than 80 million copies worldwide. As a star, he was a rich man, but Mercury was not always wealthy or famous. Yet, according to friend and fellow band member Brian May, "Freddie always looked like a star and acted like a star even when he was penniless."[2]

Freddie was born Frederick Bulsara on September 5, 1946. His family lived on the African island of Zanzibar, where his father worked for the British government. At the age of seven, Freddie was sent to boarding school in Bombay, India. The Bulsaras moved to England when Freddie was in his teens, and he transferred to a boarding school there.

During his youth, Freddie studied classical music for four years. He played the piano and often composed his own music. He liked listening to other kinds of music, too, and singer Liza Minelli became a favorite.

Freddie's idol was Jimi Hendrix. Freddie admired his music as well as his electrifying stage presence. Of Hendrix, Freddie once said, "I scoured the countryside to see him. He really had everything a rock and roll star should have. . . . He'd just make an entrance and the whole place would be on fire. He was living out everything I wanted to be."[3]

After high school, Freddie spent four years at a London art college earning a degree in graphic design and illustration. His musical interests never waned, though, and he joined small, semiprofessional bands which played in clubs around London.

In the early 1970s, Freddie convinced two musicians—guitarist Brian May and drummer Roger Taylor—to join him in creating a new band. A final member, bass player John Deacon, was recruited through a classified advertisement in a newspaper.

In 1971, Freddie named this new band Queen. He renamed himself at about this time, too, changing his last name to Mercury after the mythical messenger of the gods. Mercury, Freddie felt, was a name that suited a rock star.

Although interested in music, Queen's members were also dedicated to getting their educations. Mercury already had his degree in art, but the rest continued their schooling—Taylor studied biology, May was a graduate student in astronomy, and Deacon studied electronics. In their free time, the group rehearsed in private.

As the band practiced, Queen developed a unique style, a sound one reviewer described as a "hybrid of hard rock, pop, heavy-metal, cabaret and a hint of opera."[4] Gradually, Mercury emerged as the group's lead singer, songwriter, and pianist.

In 1973, Queen released its first album. It flopped, but the group persevered. When the band's second album hit the top ten on the British rock charts in 1974, Queen was an English success. It was Queen's third album that made the group popular in America.

As time passed, Queen's music grew more complex. Each album was an elaborate studio production that overdubbed voices and instruments. By overdubbing, the four band members could produce songs that sounded as if they were being played by an entire orchestra.

In person, Queen was also unique. Concerts were carefully calculated to include a dazzling array of special effects. Each Queen performance required a team of technicians to coordinate smoke generators, bubble-blowing machines, and flashing lights. Explaining Queen's philosophy, May said, "People are giving you two hours of their time, so you have to give them *everything* for those two hours. We want every person to go away feeling he got his money's worth, and we use every possible device to achieve that."[5]

But the biggest draw to a Queen concert was Freddie Mercury himself. Mercury, a flamboyant performer, strutted about the stage commanding the audience's attention. As one writer put it, he "projected his personality at about thirty decibels above outrageous."[6] In the course of a concert, Mercury might change his clothing several times, and his costumes ranged from the bizarre to the eccentric. It was not unusual for him to appear in chain mail, hot pants, sequined suits, military uniforms, leotards, or kimonos. Of him, rock king David Bowie said, "Freddie took it further than the rest. He took it over the edge. And of course, I always admired a man who wears tights."[7] During the late 1970s, Queen concerts packed stadiums with fans devoted to the group's slender, five-foot-ten-inch leader.

In 1976, a new album, "A Night At the Opera," hit the music stores. It included one of Queen's most unique and best-known songs, "Bohemian Rhapsody." Created by Mercury, the number included a spoofing segment of opera music. "Bohemian Rhapsody" gained resurgent popularity when it was featured in the hit movie *Wayne's World.*

When Mercury said in 1977 that Queen's goal was to get to the top, the group was certainly close.

"We Will Rock You" was released that year, a song that has been an audience cheer at sporting events ever since. Another 1977 hit, "We Are the Champions," lives on, too. Then came the success of a 1980 album that included the hits "Crazy Little Thing Called Love" and "Another One Bites the Dust."

However, not everyone appreciated Queen. Many found Mercury's lyrics distasteful. To those critics, Mercury defended his songs:

> [They are] just pure escapism. It's like going to see a film. People should just escape for a while, then they can go back to their problems. That's the way all songs should be: you listen to them, then discard them. . . . I don't have any messages I'm trying to get across or anything.[8]

Others found Mercury's stage antics childish. After attending one concert in which Mercury kicked over a speaker cabinet then bashed it with a microphone, one critic wrote, "The whole thing makes me wonder why anyone would indulge these creeps and their polluting ideas."[9] To this kind of criticism, Mercury replied, "What can I say? I'm a flamboyant personality. I like going out and having a good time. I'm just being me. The media pick up on certain things, and a lot of things get overexaggerated."[10]

Offstage, Mercury seemed just as outrageous. In his usual, no-holds-barred manner, he sometimes boasted of having many lovers and being bisexual. In addition, he had a reputation for throwing wild

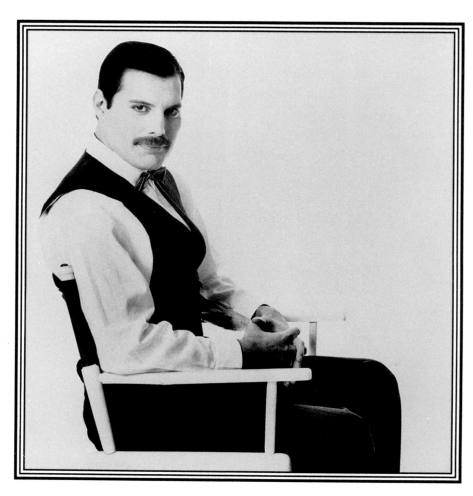

Although he was extroverted on stage, Mercury was an intensely private man. He chose to keep his illness a secret until the day before he died.

parties, which were often called "Freddie parties." At one, he swung naked from a chandelier; for another, he flew eighty friends to a resort island for fireworks and flamenco dancers.

Although no one knew it at the time, Mercury's last concert performance with Queen was in 1986. After this, he continued to record with the group, but also pursued solo projects.

Then suddenly, in 1989, Mercury dropped from sight. Without any explanation to the public, he stayed locked away in his London home. This unexplained reclusiveness led fans to believe that Mercury had AIDS. The people closest to him, however, denied this.

For two years, Mercury's friends loyally kept the secret of his illness. Then, on November 23, 1991, Mercury himself disclosed the truth—he was indeed suffering from AIDS. Through his publicist, Mercury said:

> Following the enormous conjecture in the press, I wish to confirm that I have AIDS. I felt it correct to keep this information private to date in order to protect the privacy of those around me. However, the time has now come for my friends and fans around the world to know the truth, and I hope that everyone will join me, my doctors and all those worldwide in the fight against this terrible disease.[11]

Freddie Mercury died the next day. He was only

forty-five years old. Hundreds of condolences poured in, including expressions of sympathy from superstars Elton John, David Bowie, and Ringo Starr. A small funeral service was held for Mercury's family and closest friends.

A second, more elaborate memorial was planned by the remaining Queen members. They pledged to give Mercury "an exit in the true style to which he's accustomed."[12] For this goodbye, one hundred celebrities were invited to perform in London's gigantic Wembley Stadium. On April 20, 1992, more than seventy-two thousand people gathered to celebrate the life of Freddie Mercury.

Mercury was AIDS's first victim from the rock music industry, and until his death many rock musicians had ignored the disease. Concert organizers hoped to change that. They wanted Mercury's send-off to be a commitment to the AIDS effort from rock musicians and their fans.

To that end, AIDS activists took the stage. Actress Elizabeth Taylor, who works tirelessly for AIDS research and education, spoke. Another speaker, George Michael, addressed the crowd. He told the audience that by the year 2000, more than 40 million people worldwide will be HIV-positive. He added, "If any of you really think that those are all going to be gay people or drug addicts, you're lining up to be one of those numbers."[13] As if to drive the point home, David Bowie knelt and recited the Lord's Prayer.

In addition, a myriad of musicians performed at Freddie's concert. Rock bands Metallica, Def Leppard, and Guns and Roses played. Elton John sang Mercury's famous "Bohemian Rhapsody" and Liza Minelli sang "We Are the Champions."

The concert, broadcast in seventy countries, reportedly added $35 million to the AIDS cause. This surely would have pleased Mercury, who before his death had donated a large amount of money to help AIDS projects.

It probably also would have pleased Mercury to see some of his favorite musicians gathered to pay him the ultimate tribute by singing his songs. Although the superstars performed well, some fans felt that none of them produced the same electricity that Mercury could create. As one writer put it, "It was good . . . but it just wasn't Freddie."[14]

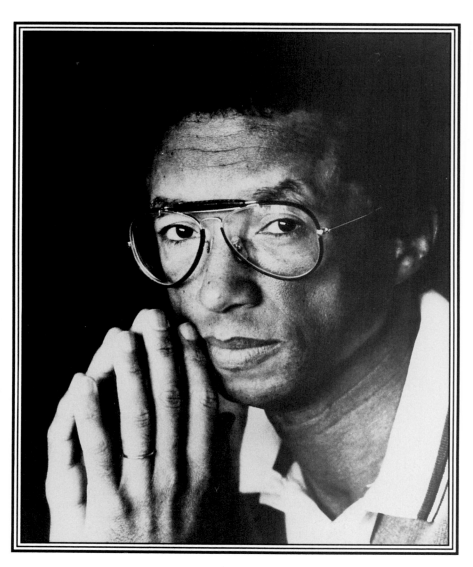

Arthur Ashe

# Arthur Ashe
## (1943–1993)

It was the last game in the final match of the United States Open tennis tournament. Now leading 40–love, Arthur Ashe let loose a powerful serve, but his opponent, Tom Okker, managed to return it. Instinctively, Ashe reached out, punched the ball past Okker, and the game was over. Ashe had won the 1968 U.S. Open!

As champion, Ashe was the first African-American man to win a world-class tennis event, but Ashe was used to being a pioneer. Since his youth, he had often been the sole African-American player on courts around the country. After this victory, Ashe continued to knock down racial barriers, opening doors for those who came after him.

Born on July 10, 1943, Arthur Ashe entered a

world he was instrumental in changing. Arthur Robert Ashe, Jr., was the first child of Arthur and Mattie Ashe of Richmond, Virginia. His father was a special policeman in charge of Brook Field, a park for African-American people, and the family lived on the park grounds. Arthur's "backyard" included a swimming pool, baseball diamonds, and four tennis courts prophetically situated right outside the family's door.

Arthur first wandered onto the tennis courts with a racquet in his hand in 1949. The young boy had other interests, too. Before he started school, Arthur's mother taught him to read, cultivating a love of books that would last his lifetime. "Many days as a kid I'd turn on soft music and read all day," Arthur once recalled.[2]

Arthur's happy world was shattered in 1950 when his mother died after a minor surgery. He was only six years old. Arthur would think of his mother every day for the rest of his life.

As his son grew, Mr. Ashe taught him to use his best manners with everyone. Mr. Ashe also believed in the value of hard work, and after school Arthur chopped wood or did other jobs. When Arthur's chores were done, he played alone, sometimes walking to a park for white children to watch them play tennis.

Arthur watched players on his "own" courts, too. One, Ronald Charity, taught him how to play tennis. At the age of eight, Arthur entered his first tournament—and lost. However, Charity recognized Arthur's talent and introduced him to Dr. Robert Johnson, a retired tennis champion from Lynchburg, Virginia.

Johnson coached promising African-American youths each summer and invited Arthur to his "camp." Arthur spent the next several summers in Lynchburg, where Johnson expected his players to be good sports as well as good athletes.

As he grew, Arthur's game improved and his sphere of competition widened. In 1955, he won the twelve and under national black tennis championship. Then he entered tournaments for whites. Many, including those in Arthur's own town, rejected his entry, but Arthur did not let racism defeat him. He played in the tournaments in which he was allowed, and practiced relentlessly to sharpen his game.

In 1960, he moved to St. Louis, Missouri, to live with a friend of Johnson's and play tennis year round. That year, Arthur won a major tournament in which he was the only African-American player. He was thrilled.

Mr. Ashe was not as ecstatic. Although proud of his son's accomplishment, he worried that Arthur might ignore his studies. He need not have worried. Arthur graduated from high school with the highest grade point average in his class.

Because of his outstanding academic and tennis abilities, the University of California at Los Angeles (UCLA) offered Ashe a scholarship, the first it had

ever given an African-American tennis player. At
UCLA, Ashe remained undefeated his freshman
year. He credited his record to professional tennis
player Richard "Pancho" Gonzales, who practiced
with him. Although Ashe was playing excellent tennis, there were still courts where he was not
admitted simply because of his race. Ashe rarely
showed how deeply this bothered him, but after one
bout of discrimination, he angrily blurted, "What
do you want me to do, paint myself with white-
wash?"[3]

During his sophomore year, Ashe was invited to
the world-famous tennis tournament at Wimbledon
in England. He was one of only 128 men in the
world so honored. Later he was named to the U.S.
Davis Cup tennis team to represent the United
States in matches around the world. Then, at the age
of twenty-one, he won the national collegiate championship. In 1966, Ashe graduated from UCLA
with a degree in business administration.

Two years in the army slowed Ashe's rising career, but when he could, he continued building his
reputation as America's best young tennis player.
Ashe was quietly proving on the court that racial
segregation was unjust: His tennis was fantastic and
his sportsmanship flawless. Beating Tom Okker in
the 1968 U.S. Open was a victory that would always
be one of Ashe's most treasured. The win catapulted
him to fame.

Knowing that fame brought obligation, Ashe

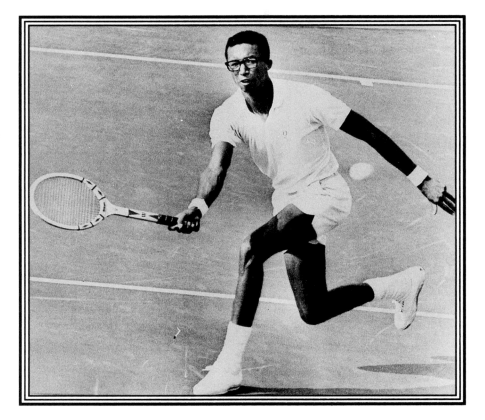

The same year Arthur Ashe won the U.S. Open, he participated in this Davis Cup match against an opponent from Spain.

became more vocal about civil rights issues. Angered by apartheid in South Africa, he led a campaign which banned that country from Davis Cup tournament play in 1970. In addition, he toured Africa in the early 1970s as a United States goodwill ambassador in support of racial integration.

Tennis was still Ashe's top priority. After a few disappointing years, he began a rigorous training program in 1975. Wanting to win at Wimbledon, the most prestigious tennis tournament in the world, Ashe entered several tournaments to ready himself. It paid off.

On July 5, 1975, Ashe stood on Wimbledon's championship Center Court facing tough competitor Jimmy Connors. As the underdog, Ashe had carefully prepared a game plan for this match, and he dominated Connors during much of the contest. When it was all over, Ashe reigned triumphant, the first African-American man ever to win Wimbledon. "When I took the match point," Ashe later said, "all the years, all the effort, all the support I had received over the years came together. It's a long way from Brook Field to Wimbledon."[4]

In 1976, Ashe achieved a major success off the court—he met New York City photographer Jeanne Moutoussamy and they fell in love. They were married in 1977.

Ashe's tennis career came to an abrupt halt in 1979 when he suffered a heart attack. Although this sudden end left Ashe temporarily bewildered about his future, he knew one thing—he would not sit still. Soon his schedule was as busy as ever. He coached the Davis Cup team and later became a tennis commentator for HBO and ABC television. He created tennis programs and mentor programs for inner-city youth and was active in causes calling for equal rights.

Health problems again interrupted his work when Ashe's heart condition called for surgery in 1983. Tragically, he was given blood during the operation that was infected with the HIV virus.[5] It would be five more years before he learned this fact.

In the meantime, Ashe's daughter, Camera, was born and she quickly became the focus of his life. As one friend said, "When [Arthur] talked about [Camera], his face would light up like stars in the sky."[6]

Now Ashe was busy writing a three-volume history of African-American athletes called *Hard Road to Glory*. As the work was being published in 1988, a disease called toxoplasmosis was attacking his system. Because this disease occurred frequently in people who were HIV-positive, doctors tested Ashe and found that he was carrying the virus.[7]

For a long time Ashe kept this discovery a secret. As he later said, "Any admission of HIV infection at that time would have seriously, permanently, and unnecessarily infringed upon our family's right to privacy."[8] Then, in 1992, a newspaper reporter learned that Ashe had AIDS. When Ashe was warned that the newspaper was about to publish this information, he called a press conference so he could reveal the illness himself.

Once he went public, Ashe became active in AIDS causes. He formed the Arthur Ashe Foundation, which raises money for AIDS research. He spoke to students and other groups across America about AIDS. Always, his message was the same. "AIDS is here and growing both in volume and complexity . . . we must do all we can to defeat it."[9]

In 1993, Ashe's health began to deteriorate. Still, he had no time for self-pity. He told a writer, "If I ask 'Why me?' about my troubles, I would have to ask 'Why me?' about my blessings. Why my winning Wimbledon? And why me marrying a beautiful, gifted woman and having a wonderful child?"[10]

To Ashe, the hardest part about dying was leaving Camera. "It's tough to understand that I won't always be around for Camera," he said.[11] He wanted to see her first communion, attend her high school graduation, and give her away in marriage.

When one reporter asked Ashe if AIDS was the biggest burden in his life, he replied, "No . . . being black is the greatest burden I've had to bear. Having to live as a minority in America. Even now it continues to feel like an extra weight tied around me."[12]

In February of 1993, Ashe became seriously ill with pneumonia. He died on February 6, but the legacy of Arthur Ashe lives on. As one young African-American tennis player said, "Arthur showed you what is possible to be accomplished. I always wanted to follow in his footsteps and nobody can forget that he made the footsteps."[13]

After Ashe's death, his wife, Jeanne, wrote a book called *Daddy and Me.* She used Camera's words along with her own photographs of Camera and Ashe to tell the story of Ashe's illness. The Ashes hoped *Daddy and Me* would help other families in the same situation. They also hoped the book would help Camera remember her father. Arthur Ashe was a man America would not soon forget, and, as one reads Camera's words, it does not seem likely that she will, either:

> Daddy is my best buddy. In the mornings he helps me get dressed for school. At night he reads me two stories before I go to sleep. Sometimes he changes the words to see if I am really listening. But I catch him and it makes me laugh! I have learned lots of things from my daddy. And one thing's for sure—I love my daddy and my daddy loves me.[14]

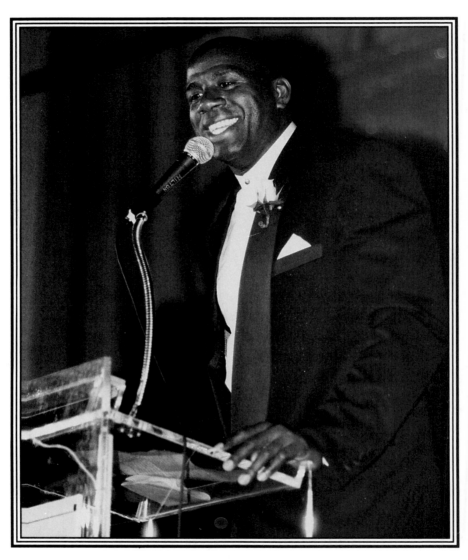

Earvin "Magic" Johnson

*When your back is against the wall, I think you just have to come out swinging. And I'm swinging . . . I'm going to go on, going to be there, going to have fun.*

—Earvin "Magic" Johnson[1]

# Earvin "Magic" Johnson
## (1959–        )

The 1979 NCAA Championship game pitted the two best college basketball players in the United States against one another—Earvin "Magic" Johnson and Larry Bird. It was a great contest, and when the final buzzer sounded, Johnson reigned victorious. He had led his Michigan State team to a 75–64 victory over Indiana State, and the Spartans were national champions! Although this game marked the end of Johnson's college career, he would go on to become a basketball legend, scoring over seventeen thousand points in twelve years of professional play.

Earvin Johnson, Jr., was born on August 14, 1959, one of Earvin and Christine Johnson's seven children. The Johnsons lived in Lansing, Michigan, where Mr. Johnson worked in an automobile factory. He also operated a part-time garbage collection business. Sometimes Mr. Johnson took Earvin with him to collect garbage, and that was when Earvin learned how to work hard. On Sunday afternoons Earvin and his father watched basketball on television together, and Mr. Johnson described the finer points of the game to his son.

Earvin did more than watch basketball. Along with his brothers and sisters, he played it on the neighborhood playgrounds. He loved the game and was on the courts after school, on weekends, and all summer long. He later said, "The courts were always packed with guys wanting to play. The only way you could hold the court was to keep winning."[2] So Earvin won.

Although much of his talent was natural, Earvin also worked constantly to improve his skills. Often he was shooting baskets by 7:30 A.M. Neighbors became so accustomed to seeing him hopping around the court that they nicknamed him "June Bug Johnson."

When he was not watching or playing basketball, Earvin was imagining entire games in his head. He sometimes fell asleep fantasizing about being a great basketball player. His parents made sure Earvin did not forget his schoolwork. Once he had to miss a championship game because he had not turned in a school assignment. His team lost without him, but he learned an important lesson.

Earvin entered Everett High School in 1974 and was soon the star of the basketball team. During one game, he racked up thirty-six points, eighteen rebounds, and sixteen assists. Writing about the contest, a local sportswriter called Earvin "Magic," and the name stuck. By his junior year in high school, "Magic" Johnson was considered one of the top high school players in the country.

Each day, he received letters from five or six colleges that wanted him to come play basketball for them. After considering his numerous options, he chose East Lansing's Michigan State University. Although the college was close and Johnson could have lived at home, he roomed in one of the school's dormitories, wanting to enjoy college life to its fullest. At Michigan State, Johnson studied and went to parties. Basketball, though, occupied a large part of his time.

Johnson was a six-foot-eight-inch freshman who played point guard—an unusual position for such a large player, but he was an excellent ball handler and he made his size an asset. During his freshman year, he led Michigan State to a 25–5 record. The next year, Johnson was instrumental in helping the Michigan State Spartans win the most prestigious title of all, the NCAA Championship.

As the premier college player in the nation, Johnson now faced an important decision. Since entering Michigan, he had been receiving offers to play professional basketball. At the end of his sophomore year, he decided he was ready to turn pro. Johnson joined the Los Angeles Lakers basketball team in 1979.

Before long, Johnson was a superstar in the National Basketball Association (NBA). Teammates and coaches credited him with having an uncanny court sense, somehow knowing where players would be before they were there. He was also a team player, willing to give shots to other teammates. Johnson's on-court statistics were impressive. At the end of his rookie season, he averaged eighteen points, seven rebounds, and seven assists a game—outstanding numbers for a guard.

The Lakers took the NBA title in 1980, and Johnson would eventually help them win four more. Johnson was voted the NBA's Most Valuable Player in 1987 and 1989. During the 1990 to 1991 season, he broke the NBA record for career assists and his record would stand until 1995. Part of what made Johnson successful was the early training from his father about the importance of hard work. Johnson once said, "I go out every night thinking I will do whatever it takes—that night—for us to win."[3]

Along with Johnson's success came fame. Everywhere the Lakers went, there were fans waiting for his autograph. Women found Johnson attractive and he was never at a loss for a female companion. Johnson made it no secret that he had sexual intercourse with many of the women he saw, but he did not become emotionally involved with any of them.

Except for Cookie. Earleatha "Cookie" Kelly was

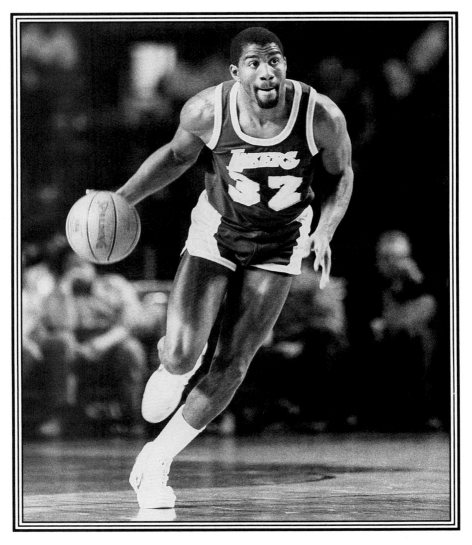

Earvin "Magic" Johnson played with the Los Angeles Lakers for his entire professional basketball career. He will long be remembered as one of basketball's all-time greats.

a woman Johnson had dated off and on since college. As time passed, he realized that he wanted her to be his wife, and in 1991 they were married.

Only weeks after the wedding, Johnson's entire life changed. His doctor stunned him with the news that he was carrying the HIV virus. Johnson had caught the disease from one of the many women he had dated before his marriage. "I was infected by having unprotected sex with a woman who has the virus," Johnson said later. "The problem is that I can't pinpoint the time, the place, or the woman. It's a matter of numbers."[4]

Telling Cookie about his illness was one of the hardest things Johnson ever had to do. She was pregnant and Johnson worried about both her and the baby because he might have passed HIV on to them. Fortunately, both have since tested negative.

Johnson's next hurdle was telling the world. "There was never any question that I would go public with this," he said. "I've always lived straight ahead, facing up to whatever happens."[5] In November 1991, Johnson made an announcement that stunned the nation. He told the public he had HIV and was retiring from basketball. Johnson explained that though he was still strong, the rigors of professional basketball might weaken his body.

Some people applauded Johnson's candor and called him a hero. Many hoped the superstar's revelation would draw national attention to the disease, along with greater awareness of its gravity. Other people did not like the idea that someone who had acted so irresponsibly should be receiving so much applause.

Johnson himself looked for a positive way to handle his tragedy. He spoke out across America about AIDS and the dangers of unprotected sex. He served on the President's National Commission on AIDS. He created the Magic Johnson Foundation, an organization to fund AIDS research, care, and education. Johnson also made time to continue his previous work with other charities such as the United Negro College Fund.

The basketball court lured him back in 1992 when Johnson joined several other superstars for the summer Olympics in Barcelona. The "Dream Team" easily captured the gold medal for the United States. Johnson also made a brief return to the Lakers as a coach and is now a partial owner of the team.

Johnson has other business interests, as well. One of his largest projects is building movie theaters and shopping centers in poor neighborhoods. Not only do these provide entertainment for the area residents, they provide badly needed jobs.

Perhaps Johnson's greatest joy is his family. Andre, Johnson's son who was born in 1981, lives with his mother, Melissa. Johnson keeps in close contact with him. In 1992, Cookie gave birth to Earvin III. The Johnsons added to their family by adopting a baby girl, Elisa, in 1995. Johnson enjoys each day he spends with his family and describes his marriage to Cookie as "the best thing that ever happened to me."[6]

When he was nicknamed "Magic" as a teenager, Johnson liked the name, saying it gave him a challenge to live up to. Now he has a new challenge—to show the world that being HIV-positive is not a reason to stop living. Johnson is optimistic and says he seldom thinks about death. He once said that he would never lose his desire to win. For Earvin "Magic" Johnson, this is as true off the court as on the court. Of beating AIDS, he says, "This is an important battle to fight—and in this battle, you are all my teammates."[7]

# Chapter Notes

## Chapter 1

1. Ryan White and Ann Marie Cunningham, *My Own Story* (New York: Dial Books, 1991), p. 256.

2. Jack Friedman and Bill Shaw, "The Quiet Victories of Ryan White," *People* (May 30, 1988), pp. 88–96.

3. Rebecca Voelker, "Ryan White, 18, Dies After 5-Year Battle With AIDS," *American Medical News* (April 20, 1990), p. 11.

4. White and Cunningham, p. 79.

5. "Breaking America's Heart," *People* (August 3, 1987), p. 61.

6. Voelker, p. 11.

7. White and Cunningham, p. 244.

8. Bill Shaw, "Candle in the Wind," *People* (April 23, 1990), pp. 86–97.

## Chapter 2

1. Steven Lee Myers, "Anthony Perkins, Star of 'Psycho' And All Its Sequels, Is Dead at 60," *The New York Times* (September 14, 1992), p. D10.

2. Brad Darrach, "Psycho II," *People* (July 13, 1983), pp. 56–64.

3. Ibid.

4. Ibid.

5. Mark Goodman, David Hutchings, and Doris Bacon, "One Final Mystery," *People* (September 28, 1992), pp. 38–43.

6. Bernard Weinraub, "Anthony Perkins's Wife Tells of 2 Years of Secrecy," *The New York Times* (September 16, 1992), pp. C15, C17.

7. Goodman, Hutchings, and Bacon, pp. 38–43.

8. Ibid.

9. Weinraub, pp. C15, C17.

10. Ibid.

11. Goodman, Hutchings, and Bacon, pp. 38–43.

## Chapter 3

1. "Notebook," *The New Republic* (March 14, 1994), p. 8.

2. David Ellis and Johnny Dodd, "Writer of Wrongs," *People* (April 26, 1993), pp. 73–76.

3. *Current Biography Yearbook*, ed. Judith Graham (New York: H. W. Wilson, 1993), p. 527.

4. William Grimes, "Randy Shilts, Author, Dies at 42; One of First to Write About AIDS," *The New York Times* (February 18, 1994), p. D17.

5. *Current Biography Yearbook*, p. 528.

6. Ibid. p. 527.

7. Garry Wills, "Randy Shilts," *Rolling Stone* (September 30, 1993), pp. 47–49, 122–123.

8. Ellis and Dodd, pp. 73–76.

9. Jerry Adler and Carey Monserrate, "And the Band Stopped Playing," *Newsweek* (February 28, 1994), p. 36.

10. *Current Biography Yearbook*, p. 525.

11. *Biographical Sketch on Randy Shilts*, March 31, 1994.

12. *Current Biography Yearbook*, p. 528.

## Chapter 4

1. Kristin McMurran and Michael Neill, "One Woman's Brave Battle with AIDS," *People* (July 30, 1990), pp. 62–72.

2. "Baby, It's OK to Go," *People* (August 24, 1992), p. 93.

3. McMurran and Neill, pp. 62–72.

4. Marianne Jacobbi, "Alison's Fight For Life," *Good Housekeeping* (September 1989), pp. 196, 246–247.

5. Bruce Lambert, "Alison L. Gertz, Whose Infection Alerted Many to AIDS, Dies at 26," *The New York Times* (August 9, 1992), p. L50.

6. Ibid.

7. Jacobbi, pp. 196, 246–247.

8. McMurran and Neill, pp. 62–72.

9. Ibid.

10. Michael Neill and Mary Huzinec, "Calm Within the Storm," *People* (March 30, 1992), pp. 59–60.

11. Lambert, p. L50.

12. "The Power of Three," *Esquire* (March 1993), p. 54.

13. Dini von Mueffling, "What I Owe My Friend Who Died of AIDS," *Glamour* (July 1993), p. 70.

## Chapter 5

1. Andrew L. Yarrow, "Keith Haring, Artist, Dies at 31; Career Began in Subway Graffiti," *The New York Times* (February 17, 1990), p. L33.

2. *Current Biography Yearbook*, ed. Charles Moritz (New York: H. W. Wilson, 1986), p. 198.

3. Michael Small, "Drawing on Walls, Clothes and Subways, Keith Haring Earns Favor with Art Lovers High and Low," *People* (November 10, 1986), pp. 52–55.

4. Ibid.

5. Paula Span, "Subways to Museums: Graffiti's Scrawl of Success," *The Washington Post* (December 30, 1985), pp. D1, D2.

6. *Current Biography Yearbook*, p. 198.

7. Ibid. p. 200.

8. Span, pp. D1, D2.

9. *Current Biography Yearbook*, p. 199.

10. David Sheff, "Just Say Know," *Rolling Stone* (August 10, 1989), pp. 58–66, 102.

11. Janice C. Simpson, "Using Rage to Fight the Plague," *Time* (February 5, 1990), p. 7.

12. Sheff, pp. 58–66, 102.

13. Yarrow, p. L33.

## Chapter 6

1. Joan Acocella, "Memories of Nureyev," *Vogue* (March 1993), pp. 356–359.

2. "Man in Motion," *Time* (April 16, 1965), pp. 48, 51–52.

3. Rudolf Nureyev, *Nureyev* (New York: E. P. Dutton, 1962), p. 39.

4. Ibid. p.42.

5. Ibid. p.52.

6. John Percival, *Nureyev, Aspects of the Dancer* (New York: G. P. Putnam's Sons, 1975), p. 25.

7. Laura Shapiro, "The Daring Young Man," *Newsweek* (January 18, 1993), p. 21.

8. "Curtain Call," *The New Yorker* (February 8, 1993), pp. 31–32.

9. Pam Lambert, "End of the Dance," *People* (November 2, 1992), pp. 60–62.

10. Jack Anderson, "Rudolf Nureyev, Charismatic Dancer Who Gave Fire to Ballet's Image, Dies at 54," *The New York Times* (January 7, 1993), p. D19.

11. Acocella, pp. 356–359.

## Chapter 7

1. Patricia McCormick, "Living with Aids," *Parents* (November, 1993), pp. 40–49.

2. Elizabeth Glaser and Laura Palmer, "In the Absence of Angels," book excerpt, *People* (February 4, 1991), pp. 83–93.

3. Geraldine Baum, "A Star in the AIDS War," *Los Angeles Times* (March 21, 1990), pp. E1, E6.

4. McCormick, pp. 40–49.

5. Ibid.

6. Elizabeth Glaser and Laura Palmer, *In the Absence of Angels* (New York: G. P. Putnam's Sons, 1991), p. 48.

7. McCormick, pp. 40–49.

8. Baum, pp. E1, E6.

9. "Messengers On Aids," *Washington Post* (August 25, 1992), pp. 6–7.

10. McCormick, pp. 40–49.

11. Ibid.

12. David Ellis, Vicki Sheff-Cahan, Kurt Pitzer, and Linda Kramer, "The Defiant One," *People* (December 19, 1994), pp. 46–53.

## Chapter 8

1. Jonathan King, "A Stilled Voice," *People* (December 9, 1991), p. 47.

2. Jeffrey Ressner, "Freddie Mercury: 1946-1991," *Rolling Stone* (January 9, 1992), pp. 13–14, 17.

3. Mick Brown, "Queen's Mercury Rising," *Rolling Stone* (May 5, 1977), pp. 11–13, 30–31.

4. "Freddie Mercury, 45, Lead Singer of the Rock Band Queen, Is Dead," *The New York Times* (November 25, 1991), p. D12.

5. James Henke, "Queen Holds Court in South America," *Rolling Stone* (June 11, 1981), pp. 41–46.

6. King, pp. 46–47.

7. Ressner, pp. 13–14, 17.

8. Henke, pp. 41–46.

9. Ibid.

10. Ibid.

11. King, pp. 46–47.

12. Kim Neely, "Freddie's Royal Send-off," *Rolling Stone* (June 25, 1992), p. 17.

13. Ibid.

14. Ibid.

## Chapter 9

1. Mary Huzinec, Maria Speidel, Rochelle Jones, and Sarah Skolnik, "Man of Grace and Glory," *People* (February 22, 1993), pp. 61–62, 68–72.

2. Ted Weissberg, *Arthur Ashe* (New York: Chelsea House, 1991), p. 26.

3. Huzinec, pp. 61–62, 68–72.

4. Weissberg, p. 23.

5. Mike Lupica, "The Righteous Rage of Arthur Ashe," *Esquire* (October 1992), pp. 101–102.

6. Huzinec, pp. 61–62, 68–72.

7. Lupica, pp. 101–102.

8. Arthur Ashe and Arnold Rampersad, *Days of Grace* (New York: Alfred A. Knopf, 1993), p. 16.

9. Ibid. p. 256.

10. Huzinec, pp. 61–62, 68–72.

11. Ibid.

12. Ashe and Rampersad, p. 256.

13. Robin Finn, "Arthur Ashe, Tennis Star, Is Dead at 49," *The New York Times* (February 8, 1993), p. B9.

14. Jeanne Moutoussamy-Ashe, *Daddy and Me* (New York: Alfred A. Knopf, 1993).

## Chapter 10

1. Keith Elliot Greenberg, *Magic Johnson, Champion With A Cause* (Minneapolis, Minn.: Lerner Publications, 1992), p. 57.

2. Bill Gutman, *Magic Johnson, Hero On and Off Court* (Brookfield, Conn.: Millbrook Press, 1992), p. 10.

3. Greenberg, p. 43.

4. Dave Anderson, "Caught In The Fast Lane," *Reader's Digest* (February 1992), p. 113.

5. Magic Johnson, "My Life," *People* (October 19, 1992), pp. 118–128.

6. Ibid.

7. Greenberg, p. 62.

# Index

H22S11536

920
GON        Gonzales, Doreen

           AIDS